Meditation as Medication for the Soul

Rajinder Singh

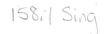

Meditation as Medication for the Soul

Rajinder Singh

Radiance Publishers

Radiance Publishers
1042 Maple Ave.
Lisle, Illinois

Publishing History
This edition first published by Radiance August 2012
Second printing: September 2012
3   5   7   9   11   13   15   14   12   10   8   6   4   2

© Copyright 2012 Radiance Publishers
Lisle, Illinois, U.S.A. 60532

Library of Congress Control Number: 2012944554
ISBN-13: 978-0-918224-72-9

Printed in Canada by Kromar Printing Ltd.

Other Books by Rajinder Singh

Spark of the Divine
Inner and Outer Peace through Meditation
Empowering Your Soul through Meditation
Silken Thread of the Divine
Spiritual Thirst
Echoes of the Divine
Spiritual Pearls for Enlightened Living
Ecology of the Soul and Positive Mysticism
Education for a Peaceful World
Visions of Spiritual Unity and Peace

In Hindi:
Spirituality in Modern Times
True Happiness
Self Realization
Search for Peace within the Soul
Salvation through Naam
Spiritual Treasures
Experience of the Soul
Spiritual Talks

Table of Contents

Part 4: Meditation for Balance and Wellness

Part 5: Meditation and the Brain

Part 6: Meditation and Pain Management

Part 7: Meditation Technique

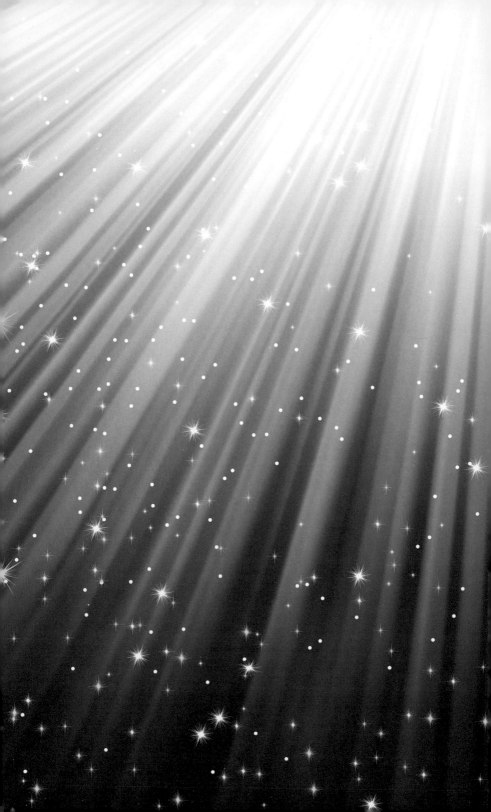

PART 1

Meditation for Spiritual Health

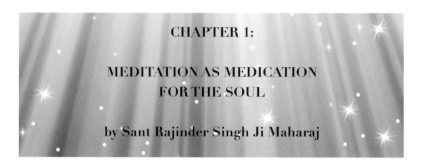

CHAPTER 1:

MEDITATION AS MEDICATION FOR THE SOUL

by Sant Rajinder Singh Ji Maharaj

Latent within each person is a spiritual energy that has the power to make us whole. The technique by which we can tap into this latent power is meditation. Once touched by this inner force we undergo a profound transformation. We experience improved health of the body, mind, heart, and soul.

In recent years, people in the West have focused attention on finding ways to heal themselves at the level of the soul to live a more fulfilling life. Many new techniques have mushroomed throughout the world.

The East offers a unique perspective. It has had a tradition for thousands of years, which the West is beginning to explore. It acknowledged a connection between the body, the mind, and the spirit. The sages of the East knew the power inherent in the soul. Western medical researchers and doctors are only recently discovering what those in the East have already known—the healing power of meditation. Medical practitioners recognize its importance. Ironically, while many in the West are employing meditation as a medical treatment, those in the East, in their quest to assimilate modern advances from the West, at times ignore their ancient traditions.

This is an exciting time to be a medical doctor. Daily, new research and medical breakthroughs astound us. Scientists and medical researchers search for cures for cancer, heart disease, strokes, and many chronic diseases. New technological tools for diagnosis, treatment, and surgery are the norm for health practitioners. They offer faster, newer, and more complex solutions, but can obscure the profound "simple" approach to wellness. Doctors can perform surgery from a remote location using robotic equipment. Tiny cameras placed in the body allow for less-invasive surgery. Body parts can be replaced in new ways. Failing hearts can now be revived. Doctors are working at the frontier of medicine.

In this dizzying array of medical innovations, meditation requires no medical equipment. Meditation is a medication for the health of the body, mind, and soul.

Meditation plays a role in preventative medicine. It has an effect on supplementing medication and speeding recovery. It has a benefit on the emotional and mental state of patients. It has a value when doctors are dealing with patients who are either terminal or who have a life-threatening illness. This book contains an array of essays on the above areas. Also, it will examine the benefits of meditation. Meditation is not meant to replace medicine or treatment, whether traditional or alternative, but is a powerful complementary tool.

Being the father of two children who graduated from medical school, I intimately know doctors, their hours, and their stress.

Doctors are a rare and noble breed. Doctors' service to humanity is beyond words. Yet, while a doctor advises patients to avoid stress, the doctor's own life itself is filled with strain. Doctors often fail to think of their own health. Meditation helps medical practitioners deal with the intense pressures of their profession. Doctors need to stay healthy for both the sake of the patients and themselves.

Meditation as Preventative Medicine

Meditation helps reduce stress, which is a normal part of life that helps the body protect itself from danger. A physical threat causes our body to release the hormones cortisol and adrenaline to provide us with the strength for fight or flight. Throughout history stress enabled people to run from an attack or to stand up to an attacker. The difficulty stress poses in modern times is that while we are seldom in physical danger from wild animals, even minor situations are perceived as mortal threats. We become stressed by events in life that we feel as earth shattering. For example, when our baby cries, we are concerned over what is wrong with him or her. If our child gets a bad grade, we worry how he or she is going to get into college. When we bring our car into a repair shop, we worry. Multi-tasking stresses us. The result is that cortisol levels flowing through our body are elevated. Cortisol might have a short-term benefit, protecting us from true physical danger, but when *everything* is perceived by our mind and body as a danger, we respond by releasing higher levels of cortisol than we need. Besides its benefits, there are dangerous side effects even when cortisone is prescribed as medicine. For example, cortisone can cause the breakdown of body tissue resulting in weakened bones and muscle tears. Thus, increased levels of cortisol and adrenaline take their toll on the body.

Medical researchers have linked certain illnesses to our state of mind and emotional condition. When we undergo mental stress, emotional pain, or depression, our physical resistance to disease drops. We become more susceptible to contracting a disease because our ability to keep our immune system in top working order decreases. Science has pinpointed heart disease, digestive problems, circulation and breathing problems, and migraine headaches to be sometimes stress-related.

Spending regular, accurate time in meditation has been shown to reduce stress. One meditation study, by Dr. John L. Craven

4

published in the Canadian *Journal of Psychiatry*, states: "Controlled studies have found consistent reductions in anxiety in meditators.... Several stress-related conditions have demonstrated improvement during clinical trials of meditation including: hypertension, insomnia, asthma, chronic pain, cardiac tachyarrhythmias, phobic anxiety." (Craven, Dr. John L., "Meditation and Psychotherapy," Canadian *Journal of Psychiatry*, pp. 648-53).[1]

In another study, Dr. Ilan Kutz states: "As the ability to meditate develops, a hierarchy of sensation develops, ranging from deep relaxation to marked emotional and cognitive alterations .... Many of these peripheral changes are compatible with decreased arousal of the sympathetic nervous system....The peripheral physiological changes have proven to be of value as a primary or adjunctive treatment for a variety of medical disorders such as hypertension and cardiac arrhythmias, as well as in relieving anxiety states and pain." (Kutz, MD, Ilan, *et al.*, "Meditation and Psychotherapy," *American Journal of Psychiatry*, Vol. 142, pp. 1-8).[2]

Meditation is a way to eliminate the lack of balance caused by mental stresses. Through it, we create a calm haven and restore our equilibrium. Researchers have recorded brain activity in people. They found that our brain waves measure from 13-20 Hz when we are involved with stressful situations at work, driving in traffic, or in a flight-or-flight mode. Those who spend time in meditation register brain waves at 5-8 Hz, a state of deep relaxation. Their mind becomes calm, which, in turn, calms the body. If we could spend some time each day in meditation, we can reduce our stress levels.

Besides reducing stress during meditation, there is a carry-over effect. We can have more inner peace of mind. As we perfect our meditations, we can maintain a calm state of mind in the midst of turmoil and strife. We can have control of our reactions and maintain an even keel.

Meditation as a Treatment Modality

In hospitals around the world, doctors suggest meditation to their patients both before and after surgery to improve their healing. With illnesses, there is pain, discomfort, and worry. When patients meditate, they can reduce the cortisol levels and aid in their recovery process. Many medical centers and hospitals routinely offer classes in meditation.

By becoming absorbed within, we can divert our attention away from the effects of illness. We come in contact with a stream of bliss and joy that takes our attention away from our pains. We enter a refuge of bliss and peace, safe from the ravages of physical pain. Meditation helps us rise above discomfort. It lifts our attention to a higher level of consciousness so that we are calm and peaceful.

Benefits of Meditation on the Emotional and Mental States

When we have an illness, it is not only the body that is in pain; our mind and emotions are often distressed. Thus, besides needing comfort of the body, we also need comfort of the mind and emotions. We live in fear of our illnesses, of what will happen to us, how we will live with any physical disabilities and limitations, what will happen to our jobs and families, and how we will pay the medical bills. There are psychiatrists, psychologists, social workers, and health care workers who are trained to alleviate fear at the mental level. There are many techniques to help people deal with their fears around their physical health. Numerous books deal with mental health and healing. Many people hold seminars on dealing with pain through coping skills at a mental and emotional level. These help bring comfort to us at a mental and emotional level. Meditation can supplement the various forms of therapy that people use to heal emotional pain. As people work on their emotional problems, often with the guidance of trained specialists, they can further increase their healing by meditating.

Meditation helps reduce emotional pain in several ways. By rising above the body, we see our lives from a clearer angle of vision. We begin to recognize the roots of our pains. Many people are not even aware of why they feel the way they do. By raising our consciousness, we become aware of the causes of our feelings.

In meditation, we come in contact with the source of all love. The current of light and sound is made of the same essence as our soul and the Oversoul. That essence is love, consciousness, and bliss. As we come in contact with it, we experience divine love. We connect with the love of God latent within us. It is said, "God is love, the soul is love, and the way back to God is through love." We may not have had love as a child and we may still be suffering from those wounds, but contact with Godly love fills that hole with more love than we can ever imagine. We can get an idea of that love by reading about the near-death experiences that people had. They describe coming in the presence of a being of light, who radiated more love to them than they ever felt in their entire lives. The love was so profound and fulfilling, many did not want to return to their body. Yet, a near-death experience just touches the border of the higher regions. Those saints and religious founders who traveled higher through meditation have described in their writings the overwhelming love they experienced. St. Catherine of Siena speaks of it as a mystic marriage with God. Mystics and saints from the East speak of union with God as an eternal marriage with their Beloved. Being drenched in that love fills the void in the heart. Thus, meditation can be an effective process for healing emotional pains.

It is noble work to bring comfort and peace to the body and mind of others. One of the greatest gifts though is comfort of the soul.

Meditation for the Soul

No matter how comfortable we make the physical body and how comfortable we make our mind, we cannot find peace until we attain comfort of the soul.

Even more poignant than the pain of the physical body, the mind, and the emotions, is spiritual pain. Within each of us, there is a deep-seated fear that cannot be soothed by physical and mental comfort. In the back of our mind, there is always the lingering fear that one day we will die. Each time this thought surfaces, we feel fear. We may have read scriptures that tell us that we have a soul that does not die, but we wonder whether it is true. In this scientific age, we have an element of doubt unless we can see for ourselves those truths. As long as we have fear, we cannot find peace. The hunger for God causes a pain deeper than any other kind. St. John of the Cross referred to it as the "dark night of the soul." We want to see our Maker, we want to know the ultimate Truth, and we want to unravel the mystery of our existence.

When spiritual hunger grips us, we begin our search. This is our spiritual awakening. We may search in our religions. We may read the scriptures, attend our places of worship, and perform rites and rituals. We may explore other religions or paths. Ultimately, when we analyze the path tread by those who found the answers—the saints, mystics, religious founders, and spiritual teachers and Masters—we come to the same conclusion, the same still point—that the way lies within and we can reach it through meditation.

The greatest comfort is peace of the soul. This only can be attained when we experience something beyond this world. That would eliminate fear of death, because we would be able to get a taste of the realms to which we will ultimately go when we depart this world. Meditation provides us such a way.

Meditative experiences are similar to near-death experiences but without the pain of nearly dying. The large Gallup poll survey taken in 1991 reported that around thirteen million people had near-death experiences. Many accounts and reports have been continuously collected revealing that this is a frequently occurring event throughout the world. It confirms the accounts of mystics, prophets, Masters, and saints through the ages. It points to a power that we can tap into when we shift our consciousness to our spiritual side. We can rise above physical pain by connecting with the power within us.

Although books on near-death experiences, or NDEs, have only been published since the 1970s, people have been experiencing this phenomenon for centuries. A typical NDE involves someone undergoing clinical death due to an accident or disease. They find themselves hovering above their body and seeing and hearing everything going on in the room. Some see medical practitioners working on their body. They see their body, with injuries and trauma, lying below them, but they no longer experience any physical pain until they return to the body. Some pass through walls and can see and hear relatives in the waiting room or even in distant cities. Suddenly, they feel themselves rushing through a tunnel and emerging at the end of the tunnel into a world of light.

Some having a near-death experience meet a being of light who embraces them with a love so fulfilling, unlike any they have ever experienced on earth. The being of light helps them through a life review in which the memories of all their thoughts, words, and deeds come back to them. Those who experience this say it is like watching a three-dimensional movie in which they are both the main character as well as the observer. They could experience the effect they had on other people throughout their lives. If they caused someone pain, then they experience the pain of others. If they brought joy to someone, they relive that as well. The people undergoing this life review come to the realization that love is the most important contribution in this world. After the review, they were told they had to return to finish out the rest of the life. They returned transformed. Realizing the importance of being loving and giving, they changed their ways. They understood that our accounts are weighed by the amount of love, service, sacrifice, and goodness, not by our money or the extent of our name and fame. What counts is how much we love and our kindness to others. When the people having the NDEs returned they realized that the secret to making the world a better place was through love. They comprehended their spiritual side.

When we meditate, we are connecting with a stream of spiritual power. Sant Darshan Singh Ji Maharaj said in a verse:

> While drinking this [Divine] Nectar, forget the sorrows of life
> and the pains of the world
> And hum songs of beauty and love.

Spending accurate time in meditation puts us in contact with an inner nectar. This spiritual power helps us forget our sorrows.

Meditation uplifts us to realms where we find the answers to our spiritual questions. We journey to those regions that await us when we leave our physical body at the time of death. Death no longer fills us with fear for we see that it holds bliss, joy, and love.

We see ourselves as soul, and know that we are drops of the Oversoul. We become all conscious. It is at that stage that our spiritual thirst is quenched. We no longer yearn for love—we become love.

Meditation to Improve the Health of Medical Practitioners

Medical practitioners often work without a break. They must begin to think of themselves. The body, mind, and spirit need time to regroup. They need to take a break and create a sacred space and time for themselves. They should hold to that time tenaciously, and make the best use of it.

What can we do in that time to give ourselves a true break? Meditation can recharge us. In meditation, the body is still. The heart rate slows down. Our body needs that relaxation time. In meditation, agitated thoughts cease for a few minutes. When our mind is still, our soul experiences joy.

One hour of meditation can give as much relaxation as four hours of sleep. Thus, fifteen minutes of meditation during our work break can give us the rejuvenation of one hour of sleep. Imagine a one-hour nap in the middle of our day. Meditation gives us that rejuvenation.

We should consider it a part of our duty to ourselves. Those fifteen minutes are our treasure. Without it, we are being stretched beyond our endurance. We need to give ourselves a chance to return to our normal equilibrium.

There is an energy that heals us. It is a healing power known as the current of light and sound. It is referred to in all the world's religions by many other names. Through meditation, we directly contact this current and reap its numerous benefits.

By becoming absorbed within, we come in contact with the healing stream.

Masters of Sant Mat or Science of Spirituality employ a meditation on inner light and sound that brings peace to the soul. The main purpose of this meditation is to help people find inner spiritual regions. There is a beyond. We are soul, and we will live beyond the demise of our body. A direct experience of the beyond can be enjoyed by each person. It is a nondenominational technique practiced by people of all faiths, cultures, and backgrounds. It is open to all. Spiritual Masters have come throughout the ages to help us experience realms beyond this physical one.

This spiritual journey takes us through different levels of inner realms. There is an astral realm filled with more light than this physical realm. There we travel in a lighter body known as an astral body. There are beautiful sights and colors in this region unseen on earth. Even more ethereal is the causal region, which is more subtle, more blissful, and more loving. It contains equal parts of matter and consciousness. From there, there is the supracausal realm, which is predominantly consciousness with a small amount of illusion. Finally, there is the region of all spirit, with no trace of matter. It is here that our soul merges into the Higher Power, called by many names in different cultures, and becomes one with the Divine. Here, we realize that our soul is of the same essence as God and is a part of God. In this state, we gain immortality, permanent peace, and divine love that knows no end. We can attain each of these states through meditation on the inner light and sound, or Shabd Meditation, as taught by Masters of Sant Mat.

In the inner realms, there is no sickness and suffering. Someone once put a sign in a newspaper that said, "House for sale in heaven. There is no mortgage to pay. We do not have to worry about electric and gas bills. The light is on all the time. The house is yours free and clear, so you do not have to work to earn a living. There is continual joy and bliss in the surroundings. No taxes to pay. No death tax because there is no death. Price of the house: priceless!"

To secure our place in these inner realms, we need to meditate daily. By stilling our mind, we can witness the inner light and sound. Thus, we lose our fear of death. We journey at any time of day or night into the spiritual realms that await us. We overcome our fear of death because we see life awaiting us beyond. People who have spiritual experiences of the beyond do not fear death because they know the bliss waiting for them.

Jyoti Meditation can easily be recommended to patients, family, or friends to supplement medical treatment. For this meditative practice, find a comfortable position, one in which you can sit the longest without being disturbed. Close your eyes very gently, just as you would when going to sleep. With closed eyes, fix your gaze at a point about eight to ten inches in front of you. As you gaze lovingly and penetratingly into the middle of what you see in front of you with closed eyes, repeat any Name of God with which you feel comfortable. This Name should be repeated mentally, with tongue of thought. Repetition of this Name will keep your mind from sending thoughts. As the Name is repeated, continually gaze into the middle of what you see in front of you. You may see flashes of light or lights of any color. You may see inner vistas. Whatever you see, go on gazing. Sit for a few minutes and enjoy the peace within.

This is a beginner's meditation. It brings peace and comfort. People who are social workers, psychologists, or psychiatrists use it with patients to promote mental healing. Many people who suffer from addictions have found relief from their addictions by tapping into a place of deep peace and joy. It is used to help reduce stress-related illnesses caused by the stress of studying for high-stakes tests for jobs or careers.

Healing the World through Meditation

Each person can become an instrument in bringing about a healing of the planet. When we become peaceful within ourselves, when our physical, mental, emotional, and spiritual pains are healed, we radiate that peace to others. We no longer are a source of conflict, but are its remedy. We no longer hurt others in thought, word, or deed. Instead, we apply balm to others' wounds.

When we rise above this world through meditation, we see the light of God in all and love all creation as one family of God. We become an agent of peace and goodwill, an ambassador of love. If each person offered their soothing presence to those with whom he or she came in contact, it would not be long before we would begin to heal the world of the scars of war and hatred. Outer peace would begin to spread worldwide.

The solution for all our pains and the world's pains is not costly. It is a free solution, available to every human being on this planet. By spending time daily in meditation, we will be in continual contact with a power that can profoundly transform our lives and those around us.

May spending time daily in meditation put you in contact with a power that can provide a medication for your soul, transforming your life and that of those around you.

Sant Rajinder Singh Ji Maharaj is an internationally-recognized spiritual Master of meditation on the inner light and sound. He is president of the Human Unity Conference and head of Science of Spirituality, a non-profit, non-denominational organization with centers in forty countries that provides a forum for people to learn meditation. He is a best-selling author whose many books, translated into fifty languages, include *Inner and Outer Peace through Meditation, Empowering Your Soul through Meditation,* and *Spark of the Divine.* He also has many CDs, DVDs, and hundreds of articles published in magazines, newspapers, and journals and has appeared on television, radio, and Internet broadcasts worldwide.

He received a B. Tech Degree in Electrical Engineering from I.I.T. (Indian Institute of Technology), Madras, India, in 1967; received an M.S. Degree in Electrical Engineering from I.I.T (Illinois Institute of Technology), Chicago, Illinois, in 1970; and was awarded a Special I.I.T. Fellowship. He had a successful twenty-year career in engineering, communications, and technology, including one of the world's leading communication companies. His accomplishments have been groundbreaking, laying the foundation for many technological innovations that have become part of standard use around the world today. For his accomplishments in the fields of peace and spirituality, he received a Distinguished Leadership Award from Illinois Institute of Technology, Chicago, Illinois.

His work in the field of science, computers, and communication has given him the ability to have a scientific approach to spirituality. He makes the science of spirituality and the practice of meditation easy for people to understand and practice for themselves. He holds meditation seminars, gives public lectures, and hosts international conferences on Human Integration and Global Mysticism, presenting his powerful, yet simple meditation on the inner light and sound to millions throughout North America, South America, Europe, Africa, Asia, Australia, and Oceania. He has also presented the benefits of meditation to medical practitioners throughout the world including the National Institute of Health, All India Institute of Medical Sciences, and universities such as Harvard University, University of California, Berkeley, I.I.T Madras (Chennai), I.I.T. Delhi, I.I.T. Mumbai, and chapters of Hospice. Many doctors have learned the meditation technique from him and use this regularly with their patients.

Civic and religious leaders have recognized his spiritual and humanitarian work with numerous awards and tributes. His life has been one continuous thread of service to humanity to bring about a world of peace, unity, and spiritual upliftment.

Sant Rajinder Singh Ji Maharaj can be contacted at Kirpal Ashram, Sant Kirpal Singh Marg, Vijay Nagar, Delhi, India 110009; Tele: 91-11-27117100; or FAX: 91-11-27214040; or at the Science of Spirituality Center, 4 S. 175 Naperville Rd., Naperville, IL 60563; Tele: (630) 955-1200; or FAX: (630) 955-1205 or visit www.sos.org.

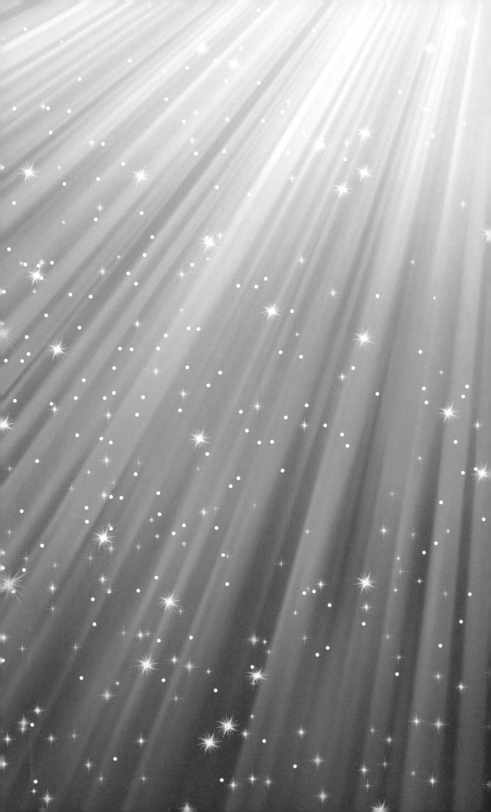

PART 2

Meditation for Physical Health

CHAPTER 2

MEDITATION: 25 YEARS EXPERIENCE IN PRIMARY CARE MEDICINE

by Matthew Raider, M.D.

Introduction

While the concept of meditation may be new to Western science, it has been practiced for not hundreds, but thousands of years. First, here are some operational definitions that will apply throughout this chapter:

Spirituality: pertaining to the spirit; the essence of each individual that is not physical and therefore not subject to deterioration

Meditation: The process whereby an individual focuses attention at a single point in an attempt to exclude distracting thoughts and outside stimuli

Health: the status of an individual physically and mentally

Healthy: the absence of disease plus the highest attainment physically and mentally of an individual given his or her inherited and environmental influences

Stress: a state of physical or mental tension; an emotionally upsetting condition occurring in response to adverse external influences be they real or perceived

For most of recorded history, little has been written about

the relationship of health and spirituality. The two were regarded as polar opposites in that health pertained to the physical body and its functions, while spirituality, if it existed outside of wishful thinking, pertained to a non-physical entity. The former was dependent on factors such as age, presence or absence of disease, environmental factors, adequate diet, and sanitation, to name but a few. This would determine if one had the features of a robust youth or a debilitated elderly person.

Science began to look at this relationship in a piecemeal fashion through some observations about meditation, prayer, and psychological adaptation in religious individuals. The study of the near-death phenomena starting in the 1970s gave a substantial impulse to the study and acceptance of the impact of meditation and similar modalities in the health arena.

Clinical Practice

When I started seeing patients in an office-based setting in 1979, I was reticent to discuss meditation or non-traditional modalities. I was practicing in a semi-rural to rural setting and the concept of meditation was largely unknown. (In 1980, I began giving lectures on meditation to the public. I would estimate that only 10% of the audience had any awareness of meditation as a technique that could be practiced by the average person.)

For the next twenty-six years, I continued to practice some general medicine, though most of my patients were over seventy, due my specialty in geriatric medicine. The office-based settings included populations from three thousand to a small city of forty thousand in central Connecticut.

Historical Perspectives

Traditional Western medicine focused on diagnosis and treatment of disease, screening for common diseases, as well as some aspects of disease prevention. It is obvious to most everyone that the explosion of technology in the 20th century resulted in tremendous advances in surgical and medical treatment of many diseases. Medications for infections, cardiac disease, cancer, asthma, diabetes, hypertension, ulcers, and many others revolutionized Western medicine in comparison to one hundred years ago. Correspondingly, surgical treatment such as bypass surgery, transplants, cataract extraction, and cancer excision to name but a few have saved millions of lives and improved the quality of many more. These advances probably led many physicians and scientists to consider only those treatments relating to "matter" as being relevant. Treatment involving prayer, meditation, homeopathy, acupuncture and other "energy" based phenomena were relegated to the irrelevant.

Meditation Physiology

In the early 1960s, Western physicians and scientists began examining meditation from the perspective of analysis. Drs. Herbert Benson and R. Keith Wallace were among the pioneers in this field.[1] Prior to this, there had been anecdotal reports of advanced meditation practitioners in India who could markedly decrease their rate of breathing.[2] Bit by bit, what emerged in the 1970s was the elucidation of meditation as a unique physiologic state with its own characteristics. It was clearly a different condition from a state of wakefulness, resting, drowsiness, hypnosis, or any of the stages of sleep. Early research corroborated the observations that regular practitioners of meditation had substantially lower respiratory rates and oxygen consumption.[3] Many changes in the body's endocrine (hormonal) responses have also been reported. Cortisol levels have been noted to decrease over the first several months after learning to meditate.[4] Cortisol (the body's natural cortisone) is produced by the outer layer of the adrenal gland (the cortex) and is the major hormone released during stress. It carries out a variety of functions vital to survival. An interesting finding has been that cortisol levels return to normal much more quickly in those who meditate regularly when compared with individuals who do not. We have all noted how our heart speeds up when we are nervous. These same researchers noted a more rapid decline back to normal heart rate in meditators. A reasonable conclusion reached from this early research is that meditation modifies the reaction of our sympathetic nervous system in a manner that appears more healthful.

There are many age-related changes in every organ system in our body. Only a few have been systematically studied with respect to being modified by meditation. The hormone dehydroepiandrosterone sulfate (DHEA-S) is produced by the adrenal gland and declines over our lifetime starting in young adulthood. An individual at age 80 will have only about one-fifth the levels they had at age 20. Dr. J.L. Glaser and associates found that experienced meditation practitioners on average have a DHEA-S level corresponding to someone 5-10 years chronologically younger than themselves.[5]

Electroencephalogram (EEG) tracings have been clearly shown to be altered. Normally, in an alert state, our EEG will show a pattern of 12-14 spikes or sharp waves per second (known by scientists as hertz or Hz). A much higher proportion of slow alpha waves were observed during meditation as well as a fairly unique pattern called theta bursts. Interestingly, theta bursts are not noted at rest or in sleep tracing of EEGs.[6] It was observed that Buddhist monks with advanced meditation practices did not flinch at the sound of a gunshot, while expert shooters will still flinch.

One measure of acute stress has been to measure what is termed skin resistance, measured as GSR, which is the basis of the lie-detector test. When stressed, skin resistance decreases. Consequently, with the exception of pathological liars, most of us are stressed when telling a fib. The effect of meditation was a marked increase in skin resistance, indicating deep relaxation.[7]

More recently, studies have utilized more sophisticated equipment, such as magnetic resonance imaging (MRI). Researchers at the University of Wisconsin and the University of Pennsylvania found significant shifts in blood flow to certain areas of the brain. Circulation to the cortex decreased, while blood flow increased in the limbic system. There was also a tendency in some areas of the brain for blood to shift from the right side to the left side.

Treating Disease with Meditation

Shortly after the research findings on meditation as being a unique physiologic state, it was but natural that attention should turn to looking at treatment of established diseases. As meditation appeared to decrease the intensity of the response of sympathetic nervous system output, hypertension was evaluated early on. Blood pressure is quite simply the pressure measured in the larger arteries of the body. It is dependent on the intensity of the heart's contractions (the pump), and the resistance the blood encounters in the arteries (the pipes). Increasingly, even mild degrees of elevated blood pressure appears to have added risk to the development of coronary disease (arteries nourishing the heart with blockages of fat, cholesterol, and blood breakdown products), heart failure (the muscular heart pump cannot pump enough blood), strokes, and less commonly, kidney failure. Dr. Benson, whose research on meditation was described above, is a cardiologist. He has stated that in the 1960s, it would have been looked at as frivolous research, so he had his subjects arrive in the off hours. He and Dr. Wallace found that by meditating regularly, individuals with high blood pressure could lower their reading by 10-12 mm of mercury, about the same as being on one blood pressure pill.[8] Their findings have been replicated by several other researchers looking at diverse populations, including young healthy individuals, the elderly, and other populations, who suffer from high rates and complications of hypertension. A recent study by Dr. R.H. Schneider published in the highly regarded American Journal of Cardiology found that meditation practice decreased the overall death rate by 23% in older persons with high blood pressure. The implication of the adoption of widespread meditation practice in hypertensive and borderline hypertensive patients is staggering. If most individuals with hypertension meditated, they could reduce their medication use by about one pill. From a financial perspective, considering the epidemic of hypertension in the United States and other Western countries, I would conservatively estimate that five billion to eight billion dollars could be saved annually in drug costs alone. The decrease in overall health costs would be many times that in all likelihood. If meditation became a universal health practice, there would be untold benefit alone from blood pressure reduction to the many individuals with undiagnosed high blood pressure and borderline hypertension. Indeed, there is even now research data to support this hypothesis.[9]

While most people fear the notion of contracting cancer more than other disease, heart disease is by far and away the number one killer in the United States. The most common form of heart disease is the slow progression of the buildup of "plaque" in the coronary arteries. These are the arteries that carry blood to the heart muscle. When one of these arteries becomes completely occluded acutely, an individual has then suffered a heart attack and a portion of the heart muscle which was nourished by that artery dies. The best hope is that a scar forms without complications and the heart still contracts normally. In the United States, this process appears to begin in late teenagers. In the Korean War, young people in the service had evidence of early plaque formation in these target arteries. In an outstanding study also published in the American Journal of Cardiology, Zamarra and his colleagues demonstrated that individuals with blockages in their coronary arteries severe enough to cause chest pain (angina) could exercise further after being "treated" with meditation.[10]

As noted earlier, many individuals with and without hypertension, often develop heart failure in middle and old age. The heart muscle either does not fill properly because it is stiff (very common in long standing hypertension) or becomes very weak and cannot contract properly. Very often, I encounter people on five to seven heart medications in an effort to maximize their poor heart function. One medication is often in the class called beta-blockers. These medications work largely by blocking the actions of adrenalin circulating in the body. In a study published in 2005, Dr. J.A. Curiati and others showed that meditation could improve the quality of life in elderly individuals with advanced heart failure. For the benefit of my scientific and medical colleagues, the enrollees in the study were taking the maximum tolerated dose of carvediol. He demonstrated lower norepinephrine (adrenalin-like) levels. I would invite my medical colleagues to review the paper as all the individuals in the trial were already on maximal medical therapy.[11] There is definitely a bias in the medical field today to use medicines and surgery as the main treatment modalities. If meditation were to come in a pill (let us call this pill "Vitamin M!"), it would already be nearly universally prescribed by cardiologists based on the studies of Drs. Zamarra, Curiati, and Schneider. Just as almost all heart patients take aspirin for its effects on preventing clots and heart attacks, it would be wonderful to see "Vitamin M" prescribed in like fashion.

Chronic pain can result from a variety of conditions and far too many are afflicted. In my current clinical practice, which includes only frail elderly individuals, I would estimate that 60% have chronic pain for which daily medicine is prescribed. Meditation has not been systematically studied for its potential benefit on a mixed population of individuals with different causes of chronic pain. One study examined individual suffering from a chronic illness called fibromyalgia. This is a syndrome that is particularly difficult to treat with traditional medication modalities. It comprises a triad of chronic diffuse pain, fatigue, and insomnia. In the experience of most physicians including myself, regular painkillers, be they mild or quite strong have a dismal record in relieving symptoms. In a study of outstanding research quality, Dr. Kenneth Kaplan and his colleagues at Boston University and Tufts Schools of Medicine enrolled 77 persons who met the strict criteria for fibromyalgia. After a ten-week program of meditation, slightly over half of those enrolled reported improvement. This is a fantastic result that should give some hope to those with chronic pain. From a research point of view, larger studies are certainly called for to see if these results can be generalized to a larger population.[12]

I am frequently asked if meditation might benefit cancer victims. This is an area where rigorous clinical trials have not yet been undertaken. There have been several observational studies, which do hold some merit. In a landmark study published in the *Lancet* (the most widely quoted medical journal in the United Kingdom) in 1989, Dr. David Spiegel reported on his findings with a group of women with terminal breast cancer. As a psychiatrist, Dr. Spiegel met with the women in a group setting twice a week and taught them a relaxation meditation technique. By his own admission, he was surprised at how long these women seemed to be surviving. After the data were analyzed, it was found that the group of women on average lived 18 months longer than would have been predicted.[13] Again, if one could bottle "Vitamin M" it would perhaps be prescribed by oncologists universally. In addition, in the study by Dr. R.H. Schneider in the American Journal of Cardiology, it was unexpectedly noted that there was a 49% decrease in the mortality due to cancer over an average of about seven years. Today, many major cancer treatment centers embrace meditation and other relaxation techniques as effective modalities.

There is a plethora of anecdotal reports that meditation helps various skin disorders. This would seem to be plausible from the vantage point that emotions and stress could certainly play a role in the most common chronic skin ailments of psoriasis, eczema, and acne. Studies have been difficult to come by and scientists do not look on case reporting as a substitute for hard evidence. One excellent study involved patients with psoriasis severe enough to be treated in a light box. This modality involves an individual being placed almost naked in a hot, noisy box while being irradiated with certain frequencies of ultraviolet light. Dr. A. Relman and colleagues had half their subjects meditate during the process. Their finding showed that the meditation group had clearing of their skin lesions at about four times the rate of the control group.[14]

There is a large amount of scientific data with respect to the benefit of meditation on mental health disorders. This is discussed at length elsewhere in this volume. Suffice it to say that meditation can be an effective modality for treatment of depression, generalized anxiety disorder, anxiety with panic, and anger management as the most common ailments. Many of us would remember that depression came somewhat out of the closet with the release of Prozac about twenty years ago. Primary care physicians were eager to prescribe it due to its better side effect profile versus older medicines, and patients found they felt so much better. Word of mouth in this case was probably far more powerful than any advertising by the drug company. Prozac was the first of drugs in a class called selective serotonin reuptake inhibitors. Translated, this means that the drug works in part by slowing the process by which the brain chemical serotonin is taken back into the brain cell. This results in higher levels of serotonin in certain brain cells. The biological theory of depression, in part, suggests that a variety of different factors may trigger lower levels of brain serotonin. These may involve severe stresses, loss of loved ones, inherited factors, and many others. At a certain point, clinicians refer to a major depressive disorder in which the brain clearly has altered levels of certain brain chemicals. It is characterized by poor mood, loss of appetite, sleep abnormalities, poor concentration, lack of interest, feelings of guilt, low energy, physical/mental slowness, and thoughts of death. Very early on, and in studies that have been verified, it was found that individuals had higher levels of brain serotonin after meditating.[15] It is no secret then that meditation can be effective for treatment and prevention of depression.

Stress

The full treatment of this topic would require an entire large volume. The research on stress and its treatment presents certain methodological problems. As one example, how does one define or even measure stress? Researchers can easily measure blood pressure, pulse, cholesterol, blood sugar, rates of heart disease, cancer, and death. How do we measure how many individuals are afflicted with stress and how severe it is? While imperfect, let us consider the operational definition given in the introduction of this article. It is my contention that stress plays a major role in

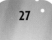

a majority of illness today and its recognition and treatment will be a major challenge in the 21st century. Given that it appears we are on target for a major financial health care crisis in the next twenty-five years, the impetus may well be financially driven.

Imagine that you find that you are in a life-threatening situation. As mammals, we are hard-wired to have a maximal "stress" reaction physically. Large amounts of adrenaline, cortisol, and other hormones pour out from our adrenal gland to act on certain organs in our body. We have probably noticed that our heart will beat fast, our mouth is dry, and we are hyper-alert. We are ready to "fight or take flight." This response has probably served mammals, including humans, quite well for millions of years. One could imagine the many circumstances in which the necessity of being at full physical and mental readiness helped sheer survival. Now, fast forward to the modern era. We are often subject to less than life-threatening stresses every week and probably every day. Instead of a massive hormonal release due to an emergency, we are getting small jolts of higher than desirable levels of cortisol, adrenaline, and other hormones. These elevated levels do their damage insidiously over months, years and decades. Simplistically, look at what happens to those who have taken large doses of cortisone (similar to the natural cortisol) for years. Cortisone was touted as the cure for arthritis several decades ago until the side effects became apparent. They often develop a moon-like face, diabetes, central obesity (large belly and chest with small arms and legs), brittle bones, muscle weakness, and other noxious effects. We have all noted what researchers have proven about short-term stress – that we are more prone to accidents, infections, and poor concentration. Over a longer period of time, many diseases appear to relate causally to elevated stress. Many studies including the author's own clinical practice suggest that stress is responsible for over half the office visits to primary care physicians. While proof is difficult to establish with certainty, a "partial" list of disorders would include alcoholism, allergies, anxiety disorders, asthma, cancer, chronic fatigue syndrome, chronic pain, constipation, depression, eating disorders, headaches (including migraine), heart disease, herpes flare up, high blood pressure, impotence, irritable bowel, peptic ulcer, sleep disorders, and smoking-related ailments. Quite a list! Just last year, Alzheimer's disease was added to that list. Dr. Robert Wilson and his coworkers at Rush Medical Center in Chicago found that those who rated their stress levels as high came down with Alzheimer's 2.4 times as frequently as compared with those with low stress levels.[16] After personally seeing over a thousand patients with Alzheimer's (and their families), this entity certainly merits our efforts to minimize the risk of contracting it. Most families I have dealt with state they would far prefer cancer to what the British term "brain failure."

Much of the research over the past few decades has been on the effects of meditation on stress. Some studies had laboratory-induced stresses such as having individuals subject to very loud horns at irregular intervals. Perhaps the most creative artificial lab stress was carried out where a group of experienced meditation practitioners and an equal number of control persons were asked to watch movies. They were told that they would see how people learned woodworking and the experiment was to measure various hormones in the subjects as they watched the movies. The researchers did not tell them that they were actually watching a group of expert stunt men and women in a mock woodworking shop. The study individuals then saw the men and women having fingers, hands, arms and legs severed off by power shop equipment, thus "stressing" them. This study and many other found that meditation had a marked attenuation of the "stress response" and that the various parameters measured such as pulse, cortisol levels, blood pressure, and adrenalin returned to baseline much more rapidly.

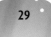

Recently, one of the biological processes as to how meditation combats stress is supported by preliminary evidence. Nitric oxide (NO) is a naturally occurring compound made in the body through some complex reactions. Dr. D.H. Kim and his colleagues found higher levels of nitric oxide production in practitioners of meditation. This reaction is thought to be one of the mechanisms by which physical damage through oxidation reactions can be prevented.[17]

Then and Now

Over twenty-five years ago, I admit that I was somewhat sheepish in "prescribing" meditation. I was an avid participant in meditation practice, but many of my colleagues and my patients thought the concept was strange. As I was a busy clinician, it was impossible to engage in rigorous research. I would talk to perhaps one patient in twenty about the potential benefits of meditation. I chose individuals whose stress was clearly distressing them. Through 1986, I was not aware of a single individual who meditated regularly based on my recommendation. In 2006, I partially retired by giving up my office practice to concentrate on teaching and nursing home medicine. In the last few years of practice, I could freely talk to anyone about meditation. About eighty percent of the patients in my practice were over seventy. The concept of meditation has become so mainstream that it appears easily accepted by nearly all. As over half my patients have stress-related disorders, it was natural to discuss meditation as a modality no different from cigarette cessation, diet management, or exercise prescription. The main drawback is that most individuals reported that they were too busy to engage in it. Approximately 10-15% of my patients towards the end of my office practice career stated they in engaged in some kind of meditation technique.

Frequently-asked Questions

After having given a few hundred lectures on the health benefits of meditation in the U.S. and Canada, the following is a short compendium of some of the more commonly asked questions:

Question: In the various studies, isn't there a difference between what technique the subjects are using?

Answer: This is an excellent research critique. In the various studies in this chapter and elsewhere, there are indeed some differences in the style of meditation, the amount the subjects meditate each day, and the length of time that the subjects have been meditating. It is clearly a major "flaw" in trying to standardize such research. This is also true of almost all the research in the area of stress as already mentioned. I do not think that this diminishes the value that these studies have provided in terms of clearly showing the benefits of meditation. It is mainly a problem of how much disease reduction, risk reduction, and potential longevity is taking place.

Question: Could the same benefit be accrued by means of bio-feedback or listening to music?

Answer: Meditation clearly has its own unique physiology and brain wave tracings. These effects were not seen during other practices such as relaxation, bio-feedback, or hypnosis. Techniques are not often compared in head-to-head studies, but I am most impressed by the studies on high blood pressure. As noted, several studies showed sustained blood pressure reduction by those continuing to meditate, which was several years in some cases. Bio-feedback seemed to lower blood pressure in the laboratory, but was harder for the subjects to reproduce on an ongoing basis.

Question: In the past, people meditated either to discover consciousness or to find God. What research is there to support any notion of consciousness or spirit?

Answer: No laboratory experiment is going to be able to answer that with certainty. There is certainly credible evidence that each individual is endowed with a non-physical essence that can survive bodily death. Let me describe an experience many years ago, not long after I received my medical degree. I was working on a Saturday and making rounds at my local hospital. One patient was a man in his late fifties who had been in the hospital for five days. He had suffered a heart attack and then a cardiac arrest while in the emergency room. The resuscitation was successful and he had been free of complications since. I walked into his room and introduced myself. After a long pause, he told me that he had left his body, but had not told anyone else thus far. He stated that he knew this was an area in which I had an interest. He had remembered everything and had watched the doctors and nurses work on him from the vantage point of floating along the ceiling. He could describe minutely how the medical equipment worked and what others were saying. He said, "I realized for the first time in my life that this body I have is only a vehicle which carries around the real me."

As this conversation took place in 1980, this man feared telling anyone as he could have been hustled off to the psychiatric unit when medically stable. Similar accounts have since been retold thousands of times. There is clearly medically credible evidence to suggest the existence of an entity (consciousness) that can function independent of the human body. I am quite fond of the later writings of Dr. Wilder Penfield, the father of modern neuroscience. After spending fifty years carrying out intense brain research, he concluded, "But the mind has energy. The form of that energy is different from the neuronal potentials that travel the axon pathways. There I must leave it."[18]

Question: I am very high strung and have a hard time sitting still. It seems like my mind is going a million miles an hour all the time. I do not think that I am cut out to meditate. Also the thought of "doing nothing" is unfamiliar to me. Isn't there something else that would help me?

Answer: While there are many relaxation techniques, the research suggests that meditation has the most powerful effects on brain and body chemistry. For someone like you, I would look at meditation as working out. When a person starts exercising, it feels onerous at first. After a few weeks, the mind seems to get in the habit of it, and one will complain if they miss their workout routine. As the mind runs in grooves, I think that if you start to meditate for even three minutes a day to start with, that would be the beginning of a habit. Every few days, you could add one minute. Within a few months, you could be meditating a half hour per day. Many people with your mental make-up report that after getting into the habit of meditating regularly, they feel something is wrong if they miss their meditation period, and report a new sense of tranquility.

Question: I have tried to meditate but I just don't have the time. What do you suggest?

Answer: Many people report that notion before starting to meditate. Many times in my medical training I was extremely busy. While in medical school I made it a point to start each day by meditating for two hours. I found that my concentration improved and I could absorb scientific material more rapidly than I could previously, and I could retain it better. This was back in 1975, and research has since corroborated the improvement in some areas of brain function in the intervening years. I think that you may find that you have more time, rather than less time, by practicing meditation.

Future Directions

I think that a paradigm shift in medicine is taking place, albeit slowly. We witnessed an explosion of medical knowledge in the last century. The challenges ahead may prove to be different from the discovery of some new pills or refining surgical technique. In all probability, we are facing a looming financial crisis in health care. When the baby boom population fully reaches retirement, we are currently ill prepared on many fronts to deal with it. Meditation has the potential to save tens of billions of dollars per year now and hundreds of billions in the future.

Research into meditation and other forms of medicine are likely to flourish. The public is deeply interested in new means of maintaining health and combating disease. Meditation would appear to offer many benefits not attainable by the standard medicinal approach. Just as regular exercise has no substitute, research should yield similar results about meditation and expand upon the current knowledge base. The current state of our understanding of brain science has to be considered still in its infancy. The unraveling of the mysteries of the brain should greatly enhance our knowledge of how meditation reprograms the brain in a positive manner.

Meditation is already mainstreamed. It could and should be prescribed universally by primary care providers as well as specialists. It can be the "Vitamin M" pill of the 21st century. Even if the phenomena cannot be fully explained as one can explain how a medication works, the success of meditation in research studies deserves a loud recommendation. I foresee primary care providers asking routinely about meditation just like cigarette cessation and exercise. Cardiologists will be prescribing "Vitamin M" along with nitroglycerin and aspirin. Psychiatrists may come to the forefront in pushing meditation for the overwhelming percentage of their patients.

I sometimes joke that I am becoming more and more like my elderly patients every day. On many days when I feel achy and tired and could use a nap, it does not seem like a joke. I imagine that as I get older, my daughters will check up on me each day to see if I have taken my pills and have meditated.

Matthew Raider, M.D. received his M.D. with honors from the University of Michigan Medical School in 1979. He completed residency in Family Medicine in 1982, during which he served as chief resident from 1981-82. Dr. Raider subsequently coordinated the geriatrics curriculum for the Middlesex Family Medicine Residency in Middletown, Connecticut, and continues to do so now. He held a faculty position at the University of Connecticut Medical School during the late 1980s in the Department of Family and Community Medicine. Dr. Raider continues to teach resident physicians as well as medical students and nurse practitioners, drawing on an extensive experience of over 150,000 patient encounters over a 30-year period. Dr Raider also has extensive expertise in the treatment of alcohol and drug dependence. He was the medical director for the Rushford Treatment Center in Middletown, Connecticut, for three years. During that time, he treated over 3,000 individuals with substance abuse problems. Currently, he is the medical director of four health care facilities in central Connecticut. Dr. Raider has long maintained an interest in meditation, vegetarian nutrition, and endurance fitness training. He has studied meditation under the guidance of Sant Darshan Singh Ji Maharaj and Sant Rajinder Singh Ji Maharaj since 1975. Matthew Raider has given several hundred lectures in the United States and Canada on the health aspects of meditation, the vegetarian diet, and the near-death experience.

CHAPTER 3

CANCER: HOW MEDITATION CAN PROVIDE A LIFELINE

by Saraswati Sukumar, Ph.D.

Professor of Oncology, Breast Cancer Program
Johns Hopkins School of Medicine, Baltimore, MD

"You have cancer." Arguably, these are the most dreaded, life-changing words that we will hear in our lifetime. But there is no denying the fact that worldwide, more than 12 million women and men are given a diagnosis of cancer each year.[1] For breast cancer alone, nearly 1.4 million new cases of breast cancer are discovered worldwide each year and nearly 500,000 women die of their disease.[2] More than 2.5 million breast cancer survivors live in the United States alone.[3] Because death rates from breast cancer are decreasing as a result of better screening, diagnosis and treatment, the number of survivors continues to increase. Although I will focus on breast cancer for the rest of my discourse, the truisms in breast cancer are easily applicable to all kinds of adult cancers.

Although the rapidity with which improvements in diagnosis and clinical care are made will never meet the expectations of those suffering from the disease and their close ones, as a researcher in breast cancer for the last thirty years, I have witnessed several seminal advancements in the management of breast cancer. Early diagnosis has led to the detection of most cancers at an early stage called ductal carcinoma in situ (DCIS), with lifetime cure rates of close to 90%. Better methods of managing the side effects of chemotherapy have made the experience less filled with fear and trepidation. A better understanding through bench research as to what has gone wrong in the tumor at the DNA level has led to some dramatic novel treatments targeting that specific mutation or change to set it right or nullify its effects. The use of Tamoxifen or aromotase inhibitors to treat women with estrogen and progesterone receptor positive (ER+/PR+) tumors and the antibody, Trastuzumab, to treat breast tumors that overexpress the gene HER2, are two dramatic examples of how research was critical to devise new treatments. As treatment gets better with each year, for many types of cancer, cancer is changing from an acute disease to a chronic one, like diabetes or heart disease. How does this translate to the number of people affected? Today, there are nearly 28 million survivors of breast cancer alone in the world.[4] For them, carrying on with life as normally as possible, despite their terrible experience and the fear of recurrence is a reality they must face. Carrying on and managing the long-term side effects of the cancer therapy their body was subjected to, is a necessity. Survivorship brings, with it, its own special needs and problems.

To understand the concepts presented in this chapter, we need to understand what is breast cancer, and what do we know about its outcome. The breast consists of 8-20 ductal trees; the trunk of each tree ends at the nipple. The entire tree is lined by an inner layer of epithelial cells and an outer layer of muscle like myoepithelial cells. Milk is produced in lobules that can be likened to flowers at the end of the branches that would look like a blossoming tree in spring. Most often, breast cancer arises from a layer of cells lining milk ducts or the lobules that supply the ducts with milk. Cancers that arise in cells lining the ducts and spread outwards are known as ductal carcinomas while those originating from lobules (the tips) are known as lobular carcinomas. Most breast cancers arise in women, but a small number of men suffer from breast cancer as well.

A number of factors go into deciding the kinds of treatment for invasive breast cancer. Treatment normally includes surgery, hormonal therapy if the tumors are hormone receptor positive or chemotherapy if they are hormone receptor negative, and radiation. Surgery alone can produce a cure in a large number of cases. To produce greater likelihood of long-term disease-free survival, several chemotherapy regimens are commonly given in addition to surgery. The major action of chemotherapy is to kill cells that are dividing rapidly anywhere in the body. Since it is not only the cancer cells that are rapidly dividing, chemotherapy often causes temporary hair loss and digestive disturbances. Radiation is indicated especially after breast conserving surgery and substantially improves local relapse rates, and in many circumstances also overall survival. In fact, survival rates across the world are generally good. Overall, more than 8 out of 10 women that are diagnosed with the disease survive it for at least 5 years.

To understand the advances that have been made in the therapy and management of breast cancer, we should look briefly at its history. How early in history was breast cancer first described, what were the treatments used, and how far have we evolved? The oldest description of cancer was that of breast cancer in Egypt and dates back to approximately 1600 BC. The Edwin Smith Papyrus described eight cases of tumors or ulcers of the breast that were treated by cauterization with the declaration that there is no treatment for the disease. Centuries passed without any innovations in the treatment. However, when doctors achieved a greater understanding of the circulatory system in the 17th century they could establish a link between breast cancer and the lymph nodes in the armpit, which allowed the tumor cells to escape to the rest of the body. This led to the removal of the lymph nodes, breast tissue, and underlying chest muscle by the French surgeon Jean Louis Petit (1674–1750) and later the Scottish surgeon Benjamin Bell (1749–1806), work that was carried forward by William Stewart Halsted at Johns Hopkins Hospitals in 1882. Halsted's radical mastectomy often involved removing both breasts, associated lymph nodes, and the underlying chest muscles, leading to long-term pain and disability. Twenty-year survival rates were only 10% before the advent of the Halsted radical mastectomy; Halsted's surgery raised that rate to 50%. For nearly 90 years, radical mastectomies remained the standard until more sparing procedures called lumpectomy were developed that proved equally effective. Modern chemotherapy developed after World War II. A number of chemotherapeutic drugs such as doxorubicin, cyclophosphamide, 5-fluoruracil, platinum derivatives and taxols are in common use. Tamoxifen and the recently developed aromatase inhibitors target ER+ breast cancers, and Trastuzumab that targets HER2+ tumors are very much in use.

A cancer diagnosis from beginning to end of successful therapy and beyond is accompanied by fear and stress. An increasing awareness of this fact has led to mind-body therapies as adjuncts to mainstream cancer treatment, and an increasing number of patients turn to these interventions for the control of emotional stress associated with cancer. Studies of mind-body interventions that include meditation and relaxation therapy, yoga, tai-chi to name some, have been shown to reduce pain, anxiety, insomnia, anticipatory, and treatment-related nauseas, hot flashes, and improved mood. Oncologists turn to research studies to provide convincing evidence that this is something they would recommend to their patients. A growing number of well-designed studies have indeed begun to provide clear evidence that mind-body techniques are beneficial additions to cancer treatment. As an article[5] in the Journal of the National Cancer Institute concluded "doctors are out there looking for things to help their patients" and studies are already easing meditation, yoga, and exercise into mainstream oncology.

One thing is certain. Having breast cancer changes your life. It not only alters your physical appearance, but more importantly, it changes how you think about your life. Fear of recurrence and death looms large. Twenty-two to fifty percent of breast cancer survivors meet the criteria for a psychiatric diagnosis of depression. Anxiety is paramount: it starts from the time of diagnosis and lasts throughout your life. Loss, grief, fear, anxiety, and loss of self-worth and self-acceptance are commonly expressed by cancer survivors. There are many potential sources of distress occurring after women have a diagnosis of breast cancer, including the diagnosis itself, anticipation of suffering, taxing treatment regimens, difficulty coping with life changes, and adjusting to the inherent uncertainty and uncontrollability of the cancer.[6] The distress diminishes breast cancer survivors' quality of life and well-being. The question is: Can one overcome or mitigate the effects of anxiety, so as to face the ordeal with equanimity but also prepare the mind in such a way that the beneficial effects are optimal while the debilitating effects can be minimized? The answer is becoming clearer by the day, and it is a firm "YES."

There is no doubt that the practice of meditation is the most effective technique for bringing the body and mind into a deep state of relaxation, restoring balance, and allowing healing to begin. Although looked upon skeptically in the beginning by the medical establishment, there is growing conviction that mind-body therapies should be used as adjuncts to mainstream cancer treatment.[6] An increasing number of patients have turned to these interventions for the control of emotional stress associated with cancer and research funds have enabled many such interventions to be evaluated for their efficacy. Is there a connection between stressed state of mind and the physiological state of the body? Can changing one alter the other?

The evidence connecting the state of the mind and its effects on physiological state of the body is incontrovertible. Stated simply, when our bodies are exposed to a sudden stress or threat, we respond with a characteristic "fight or flight" response. The hormones epinephrine (adrenaline) and norepinephrine are released from the adrenal glands, resulting in an increase in blood pressure and pulse rate, faster breathing, and increased blood flow to the muscles, to enable the body to respond accordingly. The mind experiences constant stress during the course of the disease: Have they staged my cancer accurately? Am I getting the best possible treatment? What are the right choices of treatment? What side effects will I suffer during treatment? What about after effects? How long will I live? How will my family carry on? Last, but equally important—will my insurance cover my treatment? The patient is bombarded with an overabundance of stressful situations. The distress sorely diminishes breast cancer survivors' quality of life and well-being. How does one handle this so that the mind is able to get the body in readiness to each situation so as to benefit optimally from the therapy?

Meditation is designed to elicit reactions in our body that will negate the effects of the "fight or flight" response. It is a state of deep relaxation in which our breathing, pulse rate, blood pressure, and metabolism are decreased. Meditation combined with exercise has been shown to reduce pain, anxiety, insomnia, anticipatory, and treatment-related nauseas, hot flashes, and improved mood, reduced blood pressure, heart rate, and respiratory rate.[7] Meditation affects the body in exactly the opposite ways that stress does, restoring the body to a calm state, helping the body to repair itself, and preventing new damage due to the physical effects of stress. Shielding you from chronic stress, practicing meditation allows your heart rate and breathing to slow down, your blood pressure to regain normalcy, and to use oxygen more efficiently. More importantly, the adrenal glands produce less cortisol, your brain ages at a slower rate, and your immune function improves. Your mind also clears and your creativity increases.

The meditation on the inner light and sound, which I have practiced for the last 30 years, has helped me over and over again to lead life with equanimity. Outwardly it appears that nothing stresses me out: The demands of family life, or the never-ending demands of leading a breast cancer research group. Deadlines for different grants, progress reports, seminars, and public appearances confront me with fierce determination. However, one constant companion through trials, tribulations, and happy moments has been the powerful reaffirmation provided by meditation. It provides, as a friend once told me, "the invisible fortress" or a "virtual screen of positivity" around you that deflects all negativity. This technique of meditation is a science in that the results are reproducible. Done according to the "protocol" the results are always the same. The technique is simple. We sit in a quiet place with no distracting sounds or body contact in the most comfortable position, while repeating a holy name. Gradually we lose awareness of our body, and become aware of lights of different colors and shapes and tuneful melodies. This, our spiritual teacher tells us, is the inner light and sound which we experience only when we invert our attention from our body and the impulses it constantly receives, and connect with our inner self or our soul, and feel blissful. The level of peace that you feel is an experience that permeates all the events of the day and your interactions with fellow workers and family, and makes you return to meditation faithfully every day. As my friend and fellow meditation practitioner, Dr. Mark Young, so beautifully stated in his chapter: "With the realization that we are connected to the Permanence, we gently let go of our clinging fear. We begin to glimpse that we will go on, and with that knowledge, comes courage and hope."

In conclusion, the mystery of healing remains unsolved. The quiet bliss achieved through meditation could be a powerful tool to restore normalcy to the body and strengthen the body's ability to mobilize self-repair mechanisms. A medical practice that is accepting of the power of meditation as key to rapid healing, and one that brings it into mainstream oncology, will be the hope for the future.[8]

Saraswati Sukumar, Ph.D. is the Barbara B. Rubenstein Professor of Oncology and Professor of Pathology, and a preceptor in the Human Genetics, Cellular and Molecular Medicine, Pharmacology, and Pathobiology Graduate programs at Johns Hopkins School of Medicine, Baltimore, MD. She serves as the Co-Director of the Breast Cancer Program at the Sidney Kimmel Comprehensive Cancer Center, and Principal Investigator of the NCI's Specialized Program of Research Excellence (SPORE) in Breast Cancer and of the AVON Breast Cancer Foundation. Dr. Sukumar has worked in the breast cancer field since 1978. She joined her first faculty position at the Salk Institute in La Jolla, California, in 1989, and then moved to Johns Hopkins Oncology Center in 1994 as Associate Professor and Director of Basic Research at the newly formed breast cancer research program. She was promoted to Professor in 2001. She has authored more than 140 publications. Her laboratory's work spans the entire spectrum of basic research to preclinical studies, and all the way to translation to the clinic. She was initiated into the light and sound meditation in 1972.

CHAPTER 4

MEDITATION IN THE MODERN AGE

by Kunwarjit Singh Duggal, M.D.

"Sit down and be quiet!" These were (and are) the words of my parents (Sant Rajinder Singh Ji Maharaj and Mata Rita Ji) that were reiterated several times each and every day of my life. This was easily one of the most common phrases I heard as a child growing up (understandably so as I was quite the rambunctious youth). As most children might in reaction to this statement, I would sit still momentarily before going on my energetic ways, running around, playing games, and overall causing quite the ruckus. In my novice mind, I saw this as a sign of discipline and would do my best, as many children do, to rebel against the structure and organization that would later serve me greatly in life.

Little did I know that they were giving me a gift, the best I have ever received, that would guide me in my existence as a soul on the pathway back to reunion with God, the Creator. Those five simple words provide us with the basics of meditation and allow us to begin withdrawing our attention from the physical world and channel it towards the Divine. The realization that each and every one of us are small parts of God was ingrained in me at a young age, and with the aforementioned gift I was taught and trained to access these inner spiritual realms that have allowed me to achieve a broader understanding of our existence and our goals as souls separated from their Creator.

The gift of meditation as taught by the Great Masters of Sant Mat and outlined earlier in this book by Sant Rajinder Singh Ji Maharaj allow us to ascertain our inner connection with God and experience God's grandiosity in all its glory. Surat Shabd Yoga (the form of meditation as taught by the Great Masters of Sant Mat) frees our inner consciousness from all worldly distractions, which in turn permits us to receive God in the purest form. Meditation is the forum with which we can connect with God and explore the innate spiritual essence of our beings. This spiritual awakening has guided me at each and every stage of my life: childhood, adolescence, college, medical school, and currently as a resident physician in the field of Physical Medicine and Rehabilitation.

What has become crystal clear to me over the past decade of studies and research is that the benefits of meditation are not limited to the spiritual realm. These benefits touch every aspect of our human life, be it emotionally, physically, mentally, and of course spiritually. I have seen how meditation benefits performance, mental clarity, well-being, emotional stability, health maintenance, along with health treatment and prevention.

To indulge in what may have been my first exposure to the physical benefits of meditation, I will have to take you back to the 1990s. I was an adolescent growing up in suburban Chicago. Bill Clinton was the President of the United States leading a time of economic boom. The world was in a frenzy over the Internet, a new and limitless information highway. Most importantly to me, however, was that the basketball god, Michael Jordan (MJ), was leading the Chicago Bulls basketball team to becoming perhaps the greatest sports dynasty ever created. Under the tutelage and guidance of the *Zen Master*, Phil Jackson, the Chicago Bulls went on to win six NBA championships in the span of eight years (during this time MJ took one and a half years off from basketball to pursue his childhood dream of playing baseball, accounting for the two non-championship years). It became well publicized and known throughout the sports world that Phil Jackson would often have his players meditate before games to non-pharmacologically enhance their performance. By having his players sit in silent meditation while visualizing themselves performing at the highest level, certain changes were noted: the game slowed down, shots and passes were made with an unparalleled precision, mental clarity decreased the number of mistakes and turnovers, and team play became effortless and seamless. The results were astounding: six championships with the Chicago Bulls and five more with the Los Angeles Lakers, all while dealing with some of the largest personalities in sports history while coaching Michael Jordan, Scottie Pippen, Kobe Bryant, and Shaquille O'Neil. This revolutionary system of coaching catapulted Phil Jackson above the revered Boston Celtics coach "Red" Auerbach as the consensus greatest coach in NBA history. Phil Jackson was able to get his athletes to go above and beyond their already phenomenal physical abilities by employing a technique centered on the concept of "sit down and be quiet." Did meditation give the *Zen Master* and his teams an advantage over their competitors? I believe the consensus answer is a resounding "YES!"

As an adolescent boy who loved basketball, this provided a real-life application of the benefits of meditation in the world most important to many adolescents, sports. My parents took advantage of this and would often "sell" me on increasing my meditation so I could "be like Mike." Needless to say, I spent endless hours meditating before going to shoot hoops from that point on. My meditations gave me the power to improve my concentration and mental toughness, both of which enhanced my on court abilities. The results were evident. My game did improve; however, my genetic height did not exactly keep up at the pace of my spiritual growth and my NBA dreams remained exactly that, dreams.

As I fast-forward a few years through college, medical school, and residency training, I realized increasingly the amazing effects of meditation in both the spiritual and physical realms. A recurring theme to me was the effect meditation played on stress. As you can imagine, medical school and residency training can be overwhelming at times. Urgent medical situations occur on a daily basis, and I realized the importance of keeping one's cool during these situations when trying to help those in grave danger. A common teaching in medical school training is when dealing with a code blue (emergency situation), take your own pulse before jumping in to help. This allows one to make sure they are not under too much distress that may cloud one's thinking and lead to hasty decisions in a life-and-death state of affairs. I quickly noted that I never panicked in these situations. I was able to think clearly and guide myself to make proper decisions that affected the health of those at imminent risk of death. The stress of the grave medical conditions of my patients never appeared overwhelming. My understanding of the life cycle and transmigration, with death being a sweet end to our physical existence, took away my fear of death, and this translated into what I believe is more compassionate patient care. The clarity with which I was able to think in such stressful conditions can directly be attributed to my meditation regimen. The evidence was clear to me from firsthand experience; meditation does not only lead to stress reduction in patients, but also in health care professionals, which can lead to a higher level of care for patients.

Currently hospitals employ standard-of-care treatments after extensive medical research and testing leading to *Evidence Based Medicine*. Theories are postulated and studied in animal laboratories. If successful, they are studied in small human populations, later studied in larger human populations, and after years of extensive research may or may not lead to medical discoveries that may alter the standard-of-care treatments available to greater populations. In the Western world, this leads to new pharmacological treatments that become available under the direction of an experienced physician. While this system is fantastic for medications and other therapies that are simple to study, it falters in its evaluation of practices originating in the Eastern world that are more difficult to study such as Ayurveda, traditional Chinese medicine, acupuncture, acupressure, naturopathy, homeopathy, and meditation due to the lack of standardization. These more holistic approaches to health are often tailored to each individual's lifestyle and areas of difficulty. Sworn-by practices such as these used to be often shrugged off in Western medicine with the most common argument against their support being "Where's the proof?"

Recent research has delved into these fields often with astounding results. I will focus on research in the field of meditation; however, each of these fields is now being backed with Western-world-based medical research, despite the fact that they have been routinely used throughout the Eastern world for centuries. An area of interest that particularly caught my eye deals with the benefits of stress reduction and productivity of health care workers who practiced meditation. As one can see from the following studies, the role of meditation as a practice for health care workers is crucial in providing a more optimal level of care for each and every patient, along all spectrums.

A study in the Department of Pediatrics at the University of Texas Medical branch in Galveston, Texas, employed a Mindfulness-Based Stress Reduction (MBSR) technique in academic health care employees and studied stress, various scales for health and well-being, a spiritual experience scale along with measures of pulse rate variability before, immediately after, and one year after completing an 8-week course of meditation practices. The results showed significant improvements in all measures in the group practicing MBSR immediately after the course and again one year later, while the control group (no intervention) had no significant improvements in any measures. The authors of the study concluded that MBSR effectively reduced self-report measures of stress and increased daily spiritual experiences in employees in an academic health care setting, and these effects were stable for at least one year.[1] Another study done in the Department of Surgery at the Mayo Clinic evaluated nurses before and after a month-long meditation program using computer sessions that used biofeedback to reinforce training and instruction to meditate for 30-minute sessions four times weekly for four weeks. Results showed statistically significant improvements in stress management, anxiety, and a high satisfaction with the meditation program.[2]

An Australian study at the Menzies Research Institute at the University of Tasmania focused on the effects of meditation on stress levels in their medical students. Participants underwent daily meditation for an eight-week course, and outcomes were centered on depression, stress, and anxiety. Research has established that medical students compared to the general population have higher levels of depression, stress, and anxiety. The results showed significant reductions in all fields of the study. A follow-up evaluation eight weeks after the trial ended revealed that the effects were maintained.[3] A pilot study in the School of Nursing at the City University of New York showed similar results after one month of meditation practice. Nursing student participants in this study felt calmer, more relaxed, balanced, and centered after completing the practice.[4]

What these studies show us is that it is feasible to implement meditation practices in our health care workers, and this, in turn, may lead to more complete and compassionate services for our patients. Imagine a hospital setting in which physicians, nurses, therapists, and ancillary service members are better focused, centered, rested, and compassionate. Now imagine the current state of most hospitals filled with the hustle and bustle of keeping up with administration demands, ensuring people are being discharged according to insurance mandates, and physicians and nurses being forced to "hand off" patients to ensure they do not violate strict duty hours restrictions. If given the choice, I think we would be hard-pressed to find someone willing to voluntarily accept the latter option. We have the chance to put into practice changes that will help improve patient care as we move forward. If it were my choice, I would ensure the availability and encouragement of meditation programs in health care settings, available to employees, as well as patients and their loved ones.

As a physician in the field of Physical Medicine and Rehabilitation, a physiatrist, I see a wide variety in my patient population and the ailments that distress them. The most common symptom I see in both my patients and in the general population is pain. It is one of the most basic life concepts that bind us together. Especially when dealing with chronic pain, it is necessary to give patients an assortment of modalities that may alleviate their symptoms, thus combating their symptoms on many fronts, instead of just focusing on one and hoping it works. Interestingly enough, I find that pain is one of the aspects of medicine that may be the most under and improperly treated, leaving patients with little hope. An area of interest of mine and in recent research has been the effect that meditation may make in pain modulation.

In a recent study at the Wake Forest University School of Medicine, participants underwent assessment with functional magnetic resonance imaging (fMRI) in response to pain stimulation. They were studied at baseline and again after four days of meditation training. After meditating, subjects experienced a 57% decrease in pain unpleasantness and a 40% decrease in pain intensity ratings. Using fMRI, the authors were able to note specific areas of the brain that had changes in pain-related activation directly related to meditation: contralateral primary somatosensory cortex, anterior cingulate cortex, anterior insula, orbitofrontal cortex, and the thalamus. The effect of deactivating the thalamus may reflect a change in the limbic gating mechanism that modified afferent input, essentially changing the way our brain senses pain and responds to it.[5] Another recent study in Germany also found that participants had lower pain ratings after meditating and tested with a noxious stimulus. The study also noted that meditators at baseline exhibited a higher pain tolerance than non-meditators and another group receiving electroacupuncture. A level of meditation-induced analgesia was confirmed with this study.[6]

Those in the field of chronic pain have begun to publish several significant studies on meditation's effects on pain. In a German study, women with fibromyalgia were studied before and after undergoing a structured eight-week group program teaching meditation and yoga exercises. Those practicing meditation and yoga were noted with statistically significant improvements in quality of life, pain, depression, anxiety, somatic complaints, and mindfulness.[7] Similar results were noted after a similar study in Texas on patients with fibromyalgia. Improvements were noted with pain, stiffness, anxiety, overall health status, depression, and fatigue.[8] Researchers at the Warren Alpert Medical School at Brown University studied the effects of meditation on women with chronic pelvic pain. They designed this study after noting the well-documented effects of meditation on patients with cancer pain, low back pain, and migraine headaches. After an eight-week meditation program, significant improvements were noted in daily maximum pain scores, physical function, mental health, and social function.[9] The benefits did not stop there. A recent study at Drexel University noted that meditation has noteworthy effects on pain quality of life and symptom quality of life in patients suffering from painful diabetic peripheral neuropathy.[10]

So how exactly does meditation physiologically alter our makeup to produce the beneficial changes being discussed here? The answer is becoming clearer as we speak. More and more research is being done to study specific areas of the brain that are affected by meditation. The science of spirituality is gaining evidence, and new data may help us scientifically prove observable effects of spiritual practices. An electroencephalogram (EEG) is a recording of electrical signal on the scalp, giving us insight into the activity taking place within the brain itself. A study at the Institute of Noetic Sciences in California recently performed EEG studies on people before, during, and after exposure to unpredictable outer light and sound stimuli, such as loud and frightening sounds, meant to induce a stressful state. The researchers found with EEG evidence of significant differences and concluded that while test subjects who did not meditate showed elevated stress levels, advanced meditators exhibited less stress levels. Further, the effects of meditation resulting in states of less stress continued in subjects who meditated even after the period of meditation had ended.[11] In a different EEG-based study, researchers were able to identify increased activity in the right parahippocampus gyrus, right fusiform gyrus, lingual gyrus, and inferior and medial temporal cortices. The observed brain patterns of increased activity supported the descriptions of *Samyama*, a concept from Yoga describing the contemplation, concentration, and unity involved with deeper understandings achieved via meditation.[12]

Another fMRI study on participants engaged in silent mantra meditation identified elevated activation in the bilateral hippocampus/parahippocampal formations, along with the bilateral middle cingulate cortex and the bilateral precentral cortex. This study corroborated earlier research also identifying the hippocampus as an area activated by meditation. Interestingly enough, the hippocampus is very involved with forming memories, thus identifying how meditation allows our concentration and memory to improve with practice.[13]

Even in people already suffering from memory loss, meditation can improve memory, along with the associated mood changes that go along with it. Researchers at the Jefferson-Myrna Brind Center of Integrative Medicine in Pennsylvania found that an 8-week, 12 minute a day meditation program in patients with memory loss resulted in positive changes in neuropsychological parameters, including mood, anxiety, and cerebral blood flow.[14] The division of Nuclear Medicine at the University of Pennsylvania further studied these patients using single-photon emission computed tomography (SPECT) scanning and noted significant increases in blood flow to the following areas of the brain: prefrontal, superior frontal, and superior parietal cortices. They also noted improvements in verbal fluency and logical memory.[15]

What may be even more promising are the almost immediate effects that meditation has on our cognition. According to a recent publication, a study at Wake Forest University noted that even four days of meditative practices enhanced the ability to sustain attention, mood, verbal fluency, visual coding, and working memory, reduced fatigue and anxiety, and increased mindfulness and executive functioning.[16] Evidence such as the above is very encouraging, especially in those who had not yet previously practiced meditation. Immediate effects are more gratifying and able to further promote an individual's personal drive to meditate. As any experienced meditator knows, this is a skill that requires extensive practice to improve and enhance one's experiences. While that is true, certain effects that may be experienced immediately even by novices may make the change significant enough to considerably alter their lives for the better.

The spectrum of benefits that arise from routinely practicing meditation is as broad as one can imagine. Every aspect of our life can be touched, be it spiritually, physically, mentally, emotionally, or neuropsychologically. The promising research I have shared with you is by no means a comprehensive synopsis of the evidence out there; it is simply a scratch on the surface of just how life-changing the practice of meditation can be. Jyoti Meditation, as taught by the Masters of Sant Mat, is a simple practice that can be done anywhere and by anyone. The journey to opening up one's inner eye and improving their physical being starts with five simple words, "Sit down and be quiet."

Kunwarjit Singh Duggal, M.D. has received a B.A. in Finance and a B.A. in Economics from the University of Illinois at Urbana-Champaign. He went on to receive his M.D. from Rush Medical College in Chicago, IL. He is currently in his fourth year of a residency in Physical Medicine and Rehabilitation at Rush University Medical Center. Dr. Duggal focuses on wellness using an approach combining a plant-based diet and an active, athletic lifestyle. He is also a proponent of meditation in conjunction with lifestyle changes to fight and prevent disease. Dr. Duggal is a lifelong vegetarian. He has studied meditation under the guidance of Sant Darshan Singh Ji Maharaj and Sant Rajinder Singh Ji Maharaj since 1988. He has given lectures on the health benefits of a plant-based diet, vegetarianism for an active lifestyle, medical foods and nutraceuticals, and the role of meditation in optimal health care.

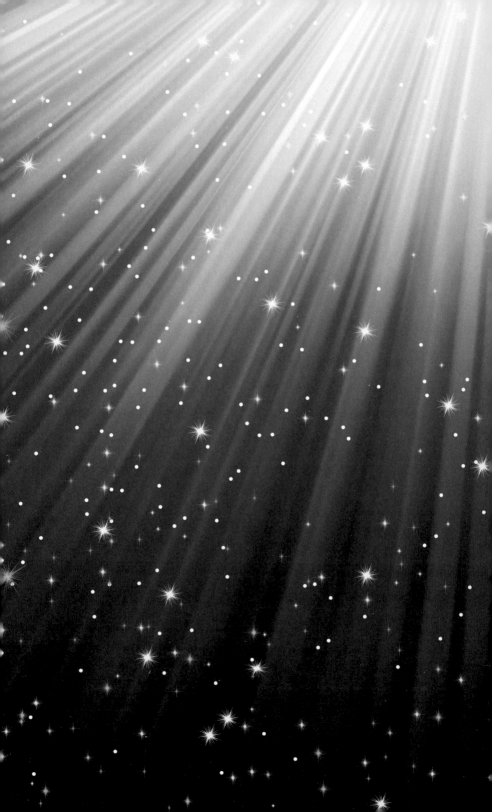

PART 3

Meditation for Mental and Emotional Health

CHAPTER 5

MEDITATION FOR EMOTIONAL WELLNESS

by Mark E. Young, Ph.D.

Professor, Counselor Education, University of Central Florida, Orlando, Florida

When my children were young, sometimes I would get annoyed or angry with them. Frequently, they would band together and say, "Dad, we think you need to meditate!" It was a good ploy to distract me from their behavior. Yet, it also reminded me of something they observed and that I had discovered as a long-time meditator: first, meditation has the effect of lowering emotional arousal during periods of stress; and second, it regulates moods, preventing angry outbursts, depressive slumps, and feelings of anxiety and fear. On the other side of the coin, meditation supports and produces positive emotions such as happiness, feelings of well-being, and joy. In other words, most experienced meditators report that they are less affected by the moods of others, accidents, and problems of the world, because of a change in consciousness that occurs as a result of their practice.

In that vein, let me tell you another story about a therapist I know who meditates. She was looking out the window and saw her client arriving at the office. As she was pouring milk into her coffee, she dropped the entire half-gallon onto the floor, creating quite a mess. She had taken a little time between clients to meditate before this accident occurred. Normally, she said, she would have gone into a series of negative mental statements such as "You are so clumsy," or "This is a horrible mess. Now I will be late for my client!" This, in turn, would have led to feelings of emotional upset. Instead, she just cleaned up the milk. Meditation helped her skip the self-defeating thoughts and emotions. No crying over spilled milk.

Meditation and a Spiritual Lifestyle to Regulate Emotions

Anger

There is a belief in some quarters that feelings of anger are healthy. Early in the last century, many counselors and therapists believed that expressing anger would lead to its dissipation like lancing a boil and letting out the poison. Now, there is a realization that expressing anger can also heighten it, while taking a toll on the physical body through the release of stress products into the blood. While there is still debate about this, many, many people who come for counseling are dealing with the consequences of anger, such as domestic violence, child abuse, poor marriage and family relationships, and problems at work, etc. Harsh words and actions damage interpersonal relationships, sometimes irreparably. These incidents are sometimes remembered for years, if not decades.

Besides angry words and actions, therapists are aware that angry thoughts are frequently the culprit in starting a spiral of anger. There is an internal dialogue a person engages in that fuels feelings of anger. One thinks of all the ways in which he or she has been wronged by another and then says to himself or herself some of the following things:

- That person should not be the way that they are.
- That person has done something mean or unjust and deserves to be punished.
- I will find a way to get even.
- I will show them they cannot treat me this way.
- It is their fault that I exploded because they made me angry.

Counselors generally believe that all of these thoughts are either demonstrably false or self-defeating. Eleanor Roosevelt said, "Nobody can make you feel inferior without your permission." Similarly, nobody can make you angry without your participation. You must be thinking one of these statements in order to work yourself into an angry state. Therapists do not believe that other people make you angry. You make yourself angry and the only person you can control is yourself. The decision to be angry takes place in a fraction of a second, but it is theoretically always preceded by one of these thoughts you have accepted. These thoughts occur automatically, but they can also be challenged and managed. Cognitive therapists challenge them on rational grounds. For example, the first statement above, "That person should not be the way that they are!" goes against reality. In fact, people are fallible and imperfect. Accepting this fact and lowering expectations of others lead to fewer feelings of hurt, disappointment, and the associated feelings of anger.

Besides the fact that these statements tend to add fuel to the emotional fire, they also have a spiritual consequence. They raise the thinker to a supposedly superior position and justify revenge because the other person has done something wrong. Anger is, in this sense, partly a consequence of an empowered ego. One seems to be saying, "If I were that person, I would not be behaving in this manner." We believe in righteous anger. Of course, the problem with that kind of thinking is that we do not understand the other person's perspective, what they have been through, whether their health is bad, or perhaps they are feeling threatened. In essence, we are suggesting that everyone ought to feel like we would in the same situation. This is the ego's inability to transcend its own viewpoint and see that others view the world differently. In my own life, I have struggled with feeling anger over wrongs committed against me. I tried to distract myself and think about other things but because I could not justify the other person's behavior, these feelings would return. I experienced daily adrenalin rushes in my body that were quite disturbing, and my attitude towards this person showed in my nonverbal behavior. When I realized that in all my thoughts about this person, I was placing myself in a morally superior position, I began examining my own behavior. I realized that I had been guilty of many of the same things as the person with whom I was angry. Thereafter, whenever one of those thoughts appeared, I reminded myself of my own behavior and that I had no right to judge that person. This had the effect of reducing my angry feelings significantly. It did not produce guilt but merely reminded me that we are all human.

Part of the spiritual lifestyle is adopting beliefs that are constructive rather than emotionally draining. What would your life be like if you did not have these negative thoughts about others and about life in general? Here are some of the ideas that spiritual seekers have tried to adopt:

1. We must change ourselves, not others.
2. There will never be a time when problems do not exist or when everyone will treat you as you think they should. We cannot entirely control the world or others. We must find peace inside.
3. What is happening to you is coming from the hand of God and is ultimately for your benefit.

What would you be feeling if you believed these thoughts instead of the nutty automatic thoughts that the ego serves up?

Dealing with Anger in the Sant Mat Tradition

The Masters of the Sant Mat tradition, which practices meditation on the inner light and sound, prescribe a daily diary of thoughts, words, and deeds. Under the *ahimsa* or non-violence category, a person keeps track of what he or she is thinking, saying, and doing with regard to anger. In addition, he or she analyzes them and tries to identify the source. By so doing, one gains insight into the thoughts that are giving rise to these deeds and actions. Ultimately, one becomes less affected by what others do because he or she does not accept the premise that the other person is wrong, villainous or malicious, and that we are always right. The Masters of Sant Mat teach that eventually anger ceases to become the automatic reaction to other people's behavior. An important point is that anger is not suppressed; it fails to surface when we really have the attitude that we do not have to take these things personally. The Sant Mat tradition teaches that conflict with others is probably unavoidable. Having different points of view is frequently helpful in identifying the most creative and effective ways to solve problems, but we need to handle the conflict in a way that does not harm others or ourselves.

Besides this long-term preventative work, the Sant Mat path recommends some emergency methods to deal with impending anger. It is suggested that taking a long cool drink of water can decrease the body temperature and prevent angry words or deeds. Similarly, it is recommended that one isolate oneself during periods of anger in order to reduce the opportunities for negative interchanges with others. Finally, having loving thoughts for others is just as important as eliminating negative ones. Finding a way to connect with others, finding avenues of agreement, and seeking harmony are antidotes to anger that are rarely recognized. Let me give you an example. When my daughter was a teenager, she and I clashed on many issues. After one difficult exchange, I made an attempt to go into her bedroom and read her a poem—something we both enjoyed. Later, I would often end the day by sitting at the foot of her bed and share a new poem with her. Poetry became a place we could easily connect and our differences did not enter in. Most of us spin our wheels by continually coming back to the part of the relationship where we disagree. Sometimes it is better to find the spot where we agree and build a relationship that will be the best medium for working through our difficulties.

As you can see, the Sant Mat tradition is spirituality in the real world. It is concerned with developing and increasing love and positive feelings in our relationships. One of the most important relationship roadblocks is anger. In order to do so, we must calm ourselves when we feel angry, prevent anger through meditation, and keep tabs on our ego, which is constantly promoting the idea that we are being persecuted by others.

Anxiety

Anxiety or fear is physiological arousal coupled with the idea that we are being threatened. Anxiety is the cause of so-called psychosomatic illness and exacerbates many other disorders. It interferes with our relationships and keeps us from enjoying life. Sometimes our fears are real. Often they are imagined or exaggerated. Either way, the body becomes aroused and a series of physiological changes occur that have been called the General Activation Syndrome. While this emergency response may help us when fleeing a burning house, the stress products in our blood can cause irreversible changes if we are merely sitting behind a desk, sweating over some paperwork. Thus, there are two kinds of stress: *physiological* and mental or *cognitive* stress. Let us say that you have just had a massage and are lying down to sleep. Physiologically, you are relaxed but your mind is chattering. The mind worries about the future or ruminates over the past. Suddenly your body is filled with tension! This example demonstrates that all of the physical exercise, hot baths, and deep muscle relaxation will not last long if we do not gain some control of our mental apparatus, which is inappropriately grinding away when we need to sleep.

Research has confirmed that there are two major ways of coping with stress: emotion-focused and problem-focused (Folkman & Lazarus, 1980). Of course, we all know that it is better to deal with problems head-on and solve them when we can rather than engage in avoidance and denial. But what about situations where there is little that we can do? Imagine that your car broke down on a lonely road and you realize that you have no cell phone and the radiator needs a mechanic. When there is little or nothing to do, we can use meditation and prayer to help us cope with the negative emotions that are causing us physical harm and clouding our thinking. Ten minutes of meditation may be enough to return us to equipoise and then we can deal with the situation in the best possible manner. This may seem like a desert island scenario but aren't there many situations in life where there is very little we can do to affect the outcome? Can we force the employer to give us the job after the interview? Can we make the professor give us a passing grade after the exam? No, but we can forestall the effects of negative emotions as we ruminate about the past or worry about the future. We can keep ourselves focused on the task at hand. If you recall my acquaintance who spilled the milk in the opening part of this chapter, we realize that meditation helps us reduce these emotions so that we can do the next thing we have to do.

Reducing Anxiety through Meditation

There is more and more convincing proof that meditators have the ability to moderate the intensity of their emotional arousal (Aftanas & Golosheykin, 2005). To illustrate this, let us look at an older study by Daniel Goleman who wrote the book called, *Emotional Intelligence* (1995). Goleman, a long-time meditator, studied meditation and stress (Goleman & Schwartz, 1976). In an experiment, he showed meditators and non-meditators films of gruesome industrial accidents. He then measured their physiological reactions to the films. Meditators were asked to meditate after the film and the non-meditators were asked to close their eyes and relax. The meditators showed a unique pattern. Like the non-meditators, they experienced the adrenalin rush of the "flight or fight" syndrome but then they rapidly recovered to their pre-film level of relaxation. On the other hand, the non-meditators reacted more slowly and continued to feel the stress both mentally and physiologically for a longer period of time. This quick stress recovery has been recognized by meditators and is a practical solution for reducing the deteriorating effects of stress as we experience a hurried lifestyle or what might be called the "full court press" of life. It seems likely that this quick recovery might also apply to other emotional challenges such as anger or sadness.

Dealing with Anxiety in the Sant Mat Tradition

Meditation brings both physical relaxation and cognitive peace that help the spiritual aspirant live with less anxiety. But the Sant Mat path also teaches us that one source of our fears is that we have all of our hopes pinned on the world as our main source of happiness. If things are going well, we are happy; if they are not, we are unhappy. We are at the whim of fate. However, what if we lived shielded from the continual ups and downs? Here, the spiritual teacher serves as a ready example of how to live life in the best possible manner. He is unaffected by roadblocks and setbacks and is happy and contented in all circumstances. He is not at all immune to the pain of others, but he is also aware of the beauty and joy of the world. This example is inspiring. We want to live in that kind of world, and the spiritual teacher assures us that it is possible. Some people object that living a life of peace and joy is somehow unnatural and that we should be affected by the slings and arrows of life circumstances. The spiritual teachers hold out the hope that if we are concentrated on God rather than the world, we will experience emotions but will not become stuck there.

Anxiety may be related to our ultimate fear—the fear of death. That is why anxiety is a spiritual issue. Although many people claim that death does not frighten them, they cringe at a lurch in an elevator or airplane. If we were not afraid of death, we would not have these automatic reactions. During meditation, the spiritual teachers tell us that we lose awareness of our body little by little. In so doing, we start to come into contact with the inner light and sound. Eventually, we realize that this experience of inner light is the light of our very own soul. Instead of thinking of ourselves as merely bodies, it slowly begins to sink in that we are eternal. As Teillard de Chardin said, we come to recognize that we are not human beings having a spiritual experience; we are spiritual beings having a human experience. With the realization that we are connected to the Permanence, we gently let go of our clinging fear. We begin to glimpse that we will go on, and with that knowledge, comes courage and hope.

Meditation and Mood

To counselors, "mood" means your general emotional state rather than a momentary period of stress or depression. This is where both meditation and a spiritual lifestyle can help. Lane, Seskevich, and Piper (2007) studied two hundred healthy adults using a number of psychological instruments that focus on mood, anxiety, and psychological distress. The clients were given a simple meditation technique and asked to practice it. Those who practiced the technique reduced both negative mood and their perceived stress. Those who practiced most frequently had the greatest effects.

While it is encouraging that meditation has an effect on negative mood, it is equally important to know that meditation can enhance moods. Frequent meditation practitioners have contended that they experience strong feelings of joy. A group of therapists (Smith, Compton, & Beryl, 1995) developed a seminar using psychological methods to increase happiness in their clients. When meditation was added to the seminar, it was found to increase significantly its effectiveness. In a related study, Wacholtz and Pargamont (2005) wanted to determine if meditation's effects on mood, pain, and anxiety were enhanced when the participants had a spiritual orientation. Participants practiced meditation for twenty minutes per day over a two-week period and then returned to the laboratory. Those with a spiritual orientation had greater decreases in anxiety, more positive mood, and could endure pain (hand in icy cold water) twice as long as the non-spiritual meditators. The research that a spiritual belief potentiates spiritual practices like meditation is growing (Benson, 1996). But spirituality is more than belief; it is a total lifestyle. Thus, benefits to our emotional wellness come from meditation, but also from how we live our lives day to day.

Dealing with Negative Moods in the Sant Mat Tradition

The spiritual lifestyle means coping with problems as they arise in the best way that you can and then leaving the rest up to the higher power. This attitude of "let go and let God," leads to a confidence and freedom from worry. Adopting this attitude has several practical steps. First, one learns to live in the living present. During meditation, one does not focus on the past and the future, and this leads to dynamic relaxation and its calming effects. You can practice this "letting go" or surrender in your daily life by focusing on what you are doing wholly and solely and not focusing on what might happen. If the task does not require mental activity, we simply try to focus completely on what we are doing rather than letting the mind wander. The mind tends to drift like the Internet surfer going from one seemingly related idea to the next and frequently finding itself lost in some unpleasant site. The Sant Mat tradition teaches that if we are fully engaged with concentrated attention on putting away the dishes, sweeping the floor, or any other task not requiring mental activity, we will not be worrying or harboring negative feelings about the past. We can use a mental repetition of God's Name to keep our consciousness focused and pay strict attention to what we are doing. During this process, our mood gradually changes to one of happiness. Below are three other aspects of the spiritual lifestyle that have an effect on our ability to deal with emotions:

1. Ethical virtues are rarely discussed as psychological tools; however, using our ethical values as an internal guidance system has clear-cut benefits. If one is acting ethically by being truthful, non-violent, loving, and humble (not believing that you are superior to others), obviously interpersonal relationships are simplified and made more peaceful.
2. Refraining from alcohol and drugs is one of the most effective

methods for reducing emotional spikes. Drugs and alcohol generally reduce inhibitions. As a marriage counselor, I have seen how things said and done during intoxication have wrecked relationships. Just as important, substances put us on a roller coaster of emotions from high to low or ease our discomfort to the place where we become inactive and avoidant. When we use alcohol or marijuana to relax, we are not learning to calm the emotions by other means. In other words, we are not practicing our coping skills but are relying on substances to forget about our stresses or dampen the pain.

3. Service to others is an important part of the spiritual path. While we are performing service, we concentrate on the task, which distracts us from negative thoughts and helps us refrain from visiting the past hurts or future worries. Yet, service also helps us get off of our ego. When we are suffering, the ego makes us believe that we alone are victims, and this can lead to feelings of depression. There is a story from Buddhism, called the "Parable of the Mustard Seed," that illustrates how focusing on others can change our attitude and feelings. A woman came to the Buddha distraught over her child's death and begged the Buddha to bring the child back to life. The Buddha said that the child could be cured with a mustard seed from a home in which no one had lost a parent, family member, or servant to death. The woman searched far and wide, but every household had suffered a loss. In her journey, she discovered that she was not unique or singled out for punishment, a belief that was prolonging her mourning.

Summary and Conclusion

The greatest benefits will accrue from those who seek guidance from a spiritual adept Science and spirituality are converging on the issue of how we can become more peaceful and happy and more in control of our own negative emotions such as anger and fear. Meditation and a spiritual lifestyle are tools that are available, without charge and without side effects. They promise better relationships, less anger, reduced anxiety and depression, more emotional stability and more positive feelings, if studied under one who is competent to guide them in their meditation practice. In addition, regular practice of meditation and a close watch on one's ethical life, including refraining from substance use, will all work inevitably to calm the waves of the emotions.

Mark E. Young, Ph.D. is Professor of Counselor Education at the University of Central Florida. For more than 20 years, he worked as a therapist in community mental health, college counseling centers, private practice, and corrections.

He is the author of five textbooks including the widely used *Learning the Art of Helping, Counseling and Therapy for Couples*, and *Counseling Today*. His research and writing has focused on wellness counseling, couples, and strength-based approaches to counseling. Dr. Young has been a state and national leader in mental health counseling and is currently President of the Association for Spiritual, Ethical, and Religious Values in Counseling, a division of the American Counseling Association (ACA). He has been honored with a number of national, state, and regional awards for his work in counseling and is a recently-named Fellow of the American Counseling Association.

CHAPTER 6

THE CREATIVE FACTOR IN SPIRITUALITY AND HEALTH

By Debbie Purdy, M.A.A.T

I open the door to my studio and immediately my mind slows down, my breathing sets a quieter pace, and my senses become more awake. Excitement to create is in the air. I have done my daily meditation practice. The stage is set for painting. I put the paper up on the wall, open the bright paints, wet the brushes, and I am off, exploring and letting the intuition and the inner stillness lead me. Colors, shapes, and images appear, and I am no longer thinking of myself. For moments at a time, there is no separation between the person and the act of creation. Creating becomes a witnessing process, where the mind takes a backseat, as the creative act takes over, allowing surprise and the unexpected. Energy comes into my awareness, along with focus and a sense of well being.

My meditation experience is similar. When I go to sit, I immediately feel a sense of quiet. I prepare by getting my meditation shawl, and turning off unnecessary noise. I fix my attention as I do in painting and go within. What arises comes from the mysterious realms of grace, outside of my control, and thrills me with a feeling of joy and love.

Creativity and spirituality are closely linked. Both lead us into the unknown. Both require a gradual process of letting go. Both require a focusing of attention that infuses us with aliveness. The creative force is that power of God going into expression. Meditation follows that power back to its original source. Being a part of a creative process helps us to bear witness to the Divine as it manifests through the force of expression. The act of creating clears the way, dumping out mental chatter, releasing unresolved issues, and integrating experiences we were not able to resolve with the mind. Meditation also stills the mind, allowing us to enter into healing realms within. Together they can partner in a mutually beneficial practice that can enhance one's inherent healing potential, engaging one's whole Self.

Meditation enables us to create with more ease from a more centered, focused wholeness of being. Creativity can help us to meditate with less confusion. Both these practices allow us to live from a place beyond the mind, which is naturally therapeutic and healing. We see that we are not our thoughts and not our feelings, that these are mere expressions that no longer define us, and we can experience a nurturing center within. While creating, an observation of thoughts and feelings can occur. We see them as flotsam and jetsam on the waves of consciousness, as we identify with the stillness that we truly are. They now have less control over our actions.

Art and creativity are wonderful ways of expressing judgments, comparisons, and concepts, in order to see them for what they are—limited and constricting thoughts that stop us. When we truly follow the process of creation, we find that we only know one part of that expression and that the spiritual wholeness within us, as it expresses through creativity, brings the larger dimensions of truth to the surface. This enables natural healing and a larger perspective, accompanied by insight, vitality, and awe.

A woman comes into a class to paint. A childhood memory arises about repression in the eastern European country of her birth. She remembers being a three-year-old asked to see if her neighbors were watching her parent's behavior. Within five minutes, her neck and shoulders are in spasms. I ask that she go to paint. She starts painting an image with the very young child and a very large adult. She sees it is her mother. Her shoulders and neck start to relax. By the end of the painting session, she is painting her mother's tears, recognizing that these tears never had permission to flow, and she is able to heal wounds that she did not know existed. Insights are coming. She no longer experiences any tension at all in her neck and shoulders, and leaves with a deep sense of well being and wholeness. This is the power of creativity to heal.

Creativity does not allow a blockage in the flow of life and attention, without signaling to us that our vital energy is slowing down. It becomes evident when tiredness, confusion, and boredom occur. Blockages are signs of judgments or fears we hold inside of ourselves, preventing the light of the attention to be fully channeled, preventing us from following our most true direction. This is also spoken of as "flow" in many books on creativity. When the flow stops, it is usually a creative block arising because of some thought.

A main benefit of imagery and creativity is integration. When events occur that overwhelm us, either emotionally or physically, the memory lodges in the body and brain, the limbic system, as trauma and, at times, body symptoms. It becomes encapsulated so as not to overwhelm the system. This experience then becomes naturally integrated through the use of imagery and art mediums. Creativity has been found to be of enormous benefit to people who have experienced traumatic events. It goes directly to the place in the brain where the memory is stored, when the whole system is ready for healing. Images arise, which then help release the disturbing event. In this way, creativity can be of help in psychological treatment. The non–verbal can cleanse the experience from our system, bypassing the logical mind, and access healing that goes beyond mental solutions.

In meditative traditions, we are asked to focus our attention. It is said that we are the attention within ourselves. If our attention is diffused throughout the body and psyche, a creative block will show us where it is. A block shows up as boredom, confusion, or fatigue. Blocks usually come from judgments or fears inside of us, preventing the light of the attention to be fully channeled. Releasing the block through the act of spontaneous creation allows the attention to flow freely and become more finely focused. This focused attention can be accessed more easily while meditating. This also has great potential for the healing capacities of creativity. New energies within the body are open for our use. These energies once unblocked, find their way to areas needing healing. Meditation also helps to refocus our attention, thus allowing us to redirect our energies to a stronger more focused spiritual experience.

Both creativity and meditation puts us into this very act of entering flow and allows the mind to be still. In the book *Flow*, by Mihaly Csikszentmihalyi, he describes how flow is the focusing of attention. He recounts neurological experiments done by Dr. Jean Hamilton, which compared experiences of students who reported either few or many flow experiences. They were given a task requiring attention and, at the same time, their cortical response was measured. Those who had reported a facility with experiencing flow in the past had a decrease in cortical activation, while those who had an infrequent experience of flow had an increase in cortical activation, more mental effort. He summarizes the data this way, "The most likely explanation for this unusual finding seems to be that the group reporting more flow was able to reduce mental activity in every information channel but the one involved in concentrating on the flashing stimuli." This can be a support of the idea that creativity helps to focus one's attention, as does meditation. He also feels that the experience of flow is where the battle for order within consciousness occurs, and that with the enhanced experience of this order a well-being is felt, accompanied by pleasure and enjoyment. This deep well-being can pervade all activities, even the most mundane. Healing occurs as the unknown part of ourselves causes integration of conflicts.

When we create, altered states naturally occur within the brain as our attention becomes focused. Cathy Malchiodi says in *The Art Therapy Sourcebook*, "The actual process of art making can alleviate emotional stress and anxiety by creating a physiological response of relaxation by altering mood. For example, it is known that creative activity can actually increase brain levels of serotonin, the chemical that is linked to depression. Other people experience art as a form of meditation, finding inner peace and calm through art expression." An active meditation takes place.

When I approach a student who is fully engaged in painting, if they are in flow, there is usually a startle response that comes about from disturbing the fine focus on the act. This also occurs when meditating. I clearly remember a time when my small son tapped me on the head when I was meditating. The reaction in my body was a startled response.

As an art therapist, I always assumed there was a connection between the spiritual and the creative. I felt that my creativity was a God-given gift. As I plunged myself deeper into the creative process, without trying to make a product or impress anyone, just following my own need for self expression, I came across the life impulse in me that was always there, sometimes coming through in meditation or spiritual connections to awakened beings. Creativity became a way of exploring that led toward that source. Meditation became the way that I would travel further along, leaving all sense of self behind. I started to use them together as a complimentary force, one opening and one going beyond. It was then that I opened a studio to share the process I had found with others. Our discussions concerning the power of creativity often included aspects of the spiritual, entering into the unknown, letting go of control, and experiencing the mystery of life. Insights, intuitions, and spiritual experiences started to flow together for participants. Painters became aware of the power of fear and judgment to stop them from experiencing their fullness, and related that to how they lived. The inner and outer life found a bridge through creativity.

Research has shown the medical benefits to the body of a meditation practice. Using states of creativity, research has also shown improvement to physical and mental health. A research study was done on Vietnam Veterans with Post Traumatic Stress Disorder, experiencing severe nightmares. They were separated into three groups. The first group was asked to sleep as usual and on awakening from a nightmare, to just note it and return to sleep. The second group was asked on waking to journal the nightmare and then return to sleep. The third group was asked to draw the images from the nightmare, and then return to sleep. Findings revealed that the first group had no change in numbers of occurrences of nightmares or severity. The second group had some improvement from writing. The third group had a huge improvement from the use of use imagery. This is a clear example of the healing powers of creativity at work. A main benefit of imagery and creativity is integration. When events occurred that have overwhelmed us, either emotionally or physically, the memory lodges in the body and brain as trauma and, at times, body symptoms. These then become naturally integrated through the use of imagery and art mediums.

Following their creative process, several of my students reported a remission of physical pain or emotional distress. One woman reported that she had had severe chronic pain for many years. As she painted, she became aware of the relationship of her own block in creativity due to the death of her sister. Her sister had died tragically at an early age and was remembered for her artistic ability. My student had blocked her creativity, thinking it was her sister's domain and somehow connected to that grief. As she let herself explore through painting, the chronic pain gradually disappeared and her grief resolved.

Another student was in the midst of a stressful career conflict at work. She experienced staff members and patrons scapegoating her, and as a sensitive person she found it hard not to blame herself. Through the creative process, she found the courage to set boundaries and release herself from the role of victim. She became less depressed and later changed jobs. She had found a sense of wholeness that instructed her without the blame, self-doubt, and criticism.

The power of creativity can be enhanced with the focus of the attention. When we bring awareness to the thoughts that might be blocking the creative flow, thoughts that are harsh, judgmental, critical, or fearful, we can notice how we are not those thoughts. A spiritual tool can be used to create from a more authentic place. We can write these thoughts on a piece of paper next to where we are creating. This is similar to using a diary to watch the thoughts that are repetitive and stop us from being present. Also, taking the time to be in the present moment, bringing the awareness back to what is in front of the artist, enhances the flow of creativity.

How does creativity work? It works in several ways. The very act of creation has powerful healing effects on the brain and body. The body is shifted to a relaxation response (similar to meditation). Hormones also shift to a healing mode. Blood flow brings in nutrients and immune cells. Neurotransmitters and endorphins reduce pain. Many report a loss of pain while creating. Within the mind, a hopeful attitude occurs. A sense of self-mastery within an internal world unfolds. Feelings of joy and peace are experienced as images are created, and the body experiences them as real. Images directly speak to the brain as the real event. Samuels and Rockwood–Lane say in their book, *Creative Healing* that an image is created, then a message is sent to the immune cells by a nerve impulse, hormone, or neurotransmitter. The cells then become activated to eat cancer cells or a virus and send blood to the area.

Images are experienced in the body as real, thus allowing disturbances to be relived and integrated and negative images in memory to be replaced by positive ones.

Meditation can also help, before a creative process. The stillness of meditation may bring one closer to the creative source. Touching those creative sources within through creativity also strengthens and nourishes the self. Through the practice of creativity, expression can occur that goes beyond the verbal. This allows a fuller expression of a thought, memory, or feeling. Add to the act of creation a few minutes of meditation and that expression can be accessed even more rapidly. At a creativity series recently, on the power of intention, the first session was started without meditation. People were asked to define intention, come up with an intention for themselves, and then make a collage using images that they cut out of magazines that resonated with that intention. The following week, the group was asked to meditate first, and as they were coming out of meditation, to allow an intention to rise up in them. They were then asked to proceed to the collage step. Most participants reported feeling free, more relaxed, and more able to find an intention that felt authentic after starting with meditation. The artwork also demonstrated a stronger sense of freedom and risk taking. If, when we create, we start from a place of diminished ego, a freer creative experience is available.

How does creativity help meditation? It helps by stilling the mind, with the release of negative thoughts. It can act as a blackboard eraser, wiping the thoughts clean before entering into meditation. One technique I use is a visual journaling process. I carry a blank journal with me, and two or three pens of different colors. When I am feeling mentally confused or distressed, I start to draw, sensing a strong point in my body and then drawing my body with a continuous line that expresses the experience within my body at different points. I do not lift up my pen. I focus more on the sense within instead of replicating the body, thus parts may be out of proportion, childlike, twisted around. I can use several colors in this drawing and it may take 5 to 30 minutes. I do not interpret or critique, but just let myself express spontaneously, letting the pen move how it wants, in any direction, feeling it in relationship to my body. Usually when I have finished, I am more relaxed, more integrated, and sometimes have an insight into the issue. This can be a good technique to use before meditation or with any kind of health challenge. At times creativity demands of us a discipline that comes out of deep longing. We are asked to go the whole way, keep working on an area, even if we do not know why. This finishing process helps us to tolerate discomfort in order to receive the rewards of full attention. We learn that we are stronger than we think, and have more stamina available to us than we know.

When we sit to meditate, we learn to tolerate the unknown and have more patience for sitting. These experiences can be fertile ground for meditation, strengthening our ability to stay still, and go beyond the everyday into an expansive wholeness of Self. Stephen Spender, the poet says, "The concentrated effort of writing poetry is a spiritual activity which makes one completely forget, for the time being, that one has a body." Creativity helps us to forget our small selves, thus experiencing the beauty of the larger unified field. This helps as we go into our meditation practice. We have a starting point, an awareness, and a possibility of going beyond the body, beyond the mind into the oneness of creation.

Thus, through experiencing creativity and meditation as active practices for healing, I have found the combination to be extremely powerful and of mutual benefit. Research has shown that creativity has direct impact on the biology of the body, which has a direct healing effect. The very act of creating for self-expression helps to unify all the inharmonious elements in the psyche that may otherwise contribute to a disease climate. Pairing a creative practice with daily meditation enhances the potential to strengthen one's immune system, by releasing stressful thoughts and encouraging a sense of well being (Samuels and Rockwood–Lane, *Creative Healing*).

Barbara Ganin says in "Art and Healing," "Psychotherapists, medical caregivers, and educators have rediscovered art as a way to heal the emotional wounds created by our internal feeling of fragmentation as well as by our sense of separation from others. Medical science has revealed that when we heal our emotional wounds, we also heal wounds of the body. As a result, art is being used successfully to reduce the physiological stress that causes immune system dysfunction."

I would encourage anyone seeking a healthier life to explore creativity and meditation as supplements to medical treatment.

I leave the studio, now. The time spent in self-expression and "flow" has put me in a rested and altered state. Insights have occurred, and I am feeling peaceful. I am ready to meditate.

Debbie Purdy, M.A.A.T. currently teaches workshops and classes on the creative process. She has a studio in Albuquerque, New Mexico, called Creative Wings Studio, and travels within the United States and abroad to teach the Creative Wings Painting Process, a process that integrates creativity and mindfulness. Before that, she had a studio in Elmhurst, Illinois, for twelve years where she did the same.

She is on the teaching staff with the founder of the process, Michele Cassou, and has been teaching with her for 12 years, in places like Esalen and The Zen Center of Los Angeles, in California, The Open Center in New York, and Zist in Munich, Germany. She holds a Masters degree in Art Therapy, which she received from the School of The Art Institute in Chicago, and a Bachelor's degree from the Rhode Island School of Design in painting. She worked as an art therapist and psychotherapist in hospitals such as Billings Hospital at the University of Chicago. She also had a private practice working in holistic centers.

Along with the Painting Process Training, other trainings were in Focusing, Hakomi, and Processwork, all leading to a deeper awareness of felt sense, as the expression of consciousness arising in the body. She has been a meditator for forty years, having been initiated by Sant Kirpal Singh Ji Maharaj.

CHAPTER 7

SPIRITUALITY AND MENTAL HEALTH

by John McGrew, Ph.D.

Since time immemorial, spiritual beliefs and practice have provided comfort to those dealing with the strife and stress of life, promising God's help in times of trouble. Faith, belief, worship, prayer, and meditation have provided spiritual succor to countless generations as they face the difficult challenges of life: suffering, illness, disability, and death. In this modern world, however, it has become fashionable to challenge and question old beliefs, often dismissing spiritual ideas or claims as myth or superstition. Whereas in the past people looked to spiritual leaders or the testimony of past spiritual masters when asking questions about why we are here and how to be happy, today, increasingly, we look to science for answers concerning our origins, health, and happiness.

Recently, however, science has begun to provide some surprising answers to what makes us happy and healthy, answers that are consistent with the teachings of spiritual traditions. For example, there is now good evidence that an active participation in a spiritual tradition may actually add as many years to your life as quitting smoking. There is evidence for the positive effect spirituality has on mental health. A growing body of evidence supports this beneficial role spirituality plays in various aspects of mental health, such as well-being, marital satisfaction, delinquency and crime, and substance abuse.

The Checkered Road to Knowledge: Mental Health and Spirituality

Through much of our history, science and spirituality have had a bumpy and at times difficult relationship. Part of the problem has been that both seek to provide answers to some of the same questions: How was the universe created? What practices heal disease? Can God heal disease? When the answers provided have differed, conflicts have arisen between science and spirituality. During the Renaissance, Cartesian dualism was proposed as a framework for a truce, relegating to science the study of the physical world and to spirituality the study of the mind or soul. However, over time, Descartes' clear division of exclusive areas of knowledge has been muddied and both science and spirituality have moved into the realm reserved for the other. The area of mental health and spirituality has been no exception. Unfortunately, conflict was the predictable initial result.

The current positive view of spirituality by psychology and psychiatry is relatively recent. Seventy-five years ago, the stance toward spirituality was most often characterized either by deliberately ignoring it or by hostility. Many early psychologists and psychiatrists believed that spiritual beliefs exerted a strong negative influence on mental health. For example, Dr. Sigmund Freud, the father of psychoanalysis, the first "talking therapy," states in his book, *The Future of an Illusion*, that religious ideas "are illusions, fulfillment of the oldest, strongest and most urgent wishes" of humanity and that the "effect of religious consolations may be likened to that of a narcotic." The founders of behavioral psychology, B.F. Skinner and John Watson, as well as Albert Ellis, one of the founders of cognitive psychology, were all vocal atheists. Suspicion of spiritual beliefs permeated the fields of

83

psychology and psychiatry, leading to a stark divide between the beliefs of scientists, psychologists, and psychiatrists on the one hand and the beliefs of their clients and the population at large on the other. For example, whereas 93% of people in the United States believe in God or a higher power (2008 Gallup Poll), and 77% believe that God can help to cure serious illness (*Time*, June 24, 1996), as many as 28% of psychologists, 21% of psychiatrists in mental health practice, and 60% of psychologists teaching at universities are atheists or agnostics.

Given these negative beliefs, it is perhaps unsurprising that some of the earliest investigations into spirituality attempted to identify *negative* effects on mental health. However, over time, a strange thing happened. The findings, instead of showing negative effects, kept showing positive ones. Scientists, reluctantly at first, eventually responded to the empirical evidence. By the end of the 20th Century, the tide had turned, so that by the 1990s the American Psychological Association published a series of influential books sympathetic to spirituality and religion. What was this evidence; why has science begun to embrace spirituality?

The Evidence for the Positive Effect of Spirituality on Mental Illness

There have been hundreds of studies examining mental health and spirituality. I will focus on the effect of spiritual belief and practice on five representative areas: well-being, marriage, delinquency/crime, substance use and psychopathology, including depression, anxiety, psychosis, and suicide. In doing the review, I relied heavily on the work of Dr. Harold Koenig of Duke Medical School and his colleagues in their book, *Handbook of Religion and Health*. In addition, although there have been some isolated findings showing an advantage of one specific set of spiritual beliefs, practices, or religion over another, the vast majority of studies fail to find differences, instead noting the importance of spirituality, regardless of the specific belief or practice. Thus, I do not review studies comparing spiritual beliefs or religious affiliation.

Well-being. Does commitment to one's spirituality produce a sense of well-being, of positive mental health? Out of 100 studies reviewed by Koenig and his colleagues, 79 yielded evidence that involvement (attendance at religious or spiritual functions and strength of spiritual or religious commitment) is associated with greater happiness and well being. For example, one study of over 6500 individuals found that 50.6% of those who attended a religious or spiritual service at least weekly were very satisfied with their lives, compared to 41.4% of those who reported no involvement. Moreover, across studies, the findings applied across every racial, ethnic, demographic, and spiritual/religious subgroup examined, including younger and older people, men and women, and people of all spiritual/religious and ethnic backgrounds. Thus, there is clear evidence that spirituality is strongly and consistently related to positive mental health.

Marital satisfaction. Does spirituality lead to greater marital happiness? Consistent with the nearly universal encouragement of marriage found in the world's scriptures, the resounding answer is yes. Thirty-five of 38 separate studies found higher marital satisfaction and lower divorce rates for persons reporting greater spiritual involvement. For example, in the United States, couples who attended their temple, synagogue, church, or spiritual meeting regularly were less likely to be divorced or separated both early in their marriage, after 5 years (7% vs. 17%), and later in their marriage, after 15 years (14% vs. 37%). A key factor underlying the lower divorce rates for these couples was an increased personal commitment to marriage, including a willingness to work through problems. However, the lower divorce rates were not due to sacrificing one's personal happiness to a sense of spiritual duty, for example, by staying in loveless marriages. In actuality, spiritually active couples have happier marriages, overall, and in studies of successful long-term marriages, the most consistently cited factors are personal spiritual belief and shared spiritual values.

Delinquency/crime. Are spiritual individuals less likely to engage in criminal activities? Certainly, the scriptures of all spiritual traditions emphasize honesty, ethical living, and respect for others. To the extent that individuals follow the teachings of their spiritual tradition, then, one would expect decreased crime among those with increased involvement, and this is exactly what the research shows. Out of 36 studies reported by Koenig and colleagues, 78% (28) reported fewer criminal activities among those with greater spiritual involvement, including decreased delinquency among youths and decreased criminality among adults. Moreover, spiritual involvement seems to lower all types of criminal activities, violent and non-violent. Interestingly, involvement in spiritual activities (e.g., attendance) was more strongly related to reduced criminal behavior than simply endorsing spiritual beliefs (e.g., belief in God). That is, in this context actions "speak louder" than words. In addition to preventing crime, spiritually-based programs may help to reduce recidivism among those already convicted. For example, inmates who attended at least 10 Bible studies were much less likely to be rearrested within one year of release (14% vs. 41%). Thus, there is clear evidence that spiritual involvement helps to reduce/prevent criminal behavior and initial evidence that it may help to rehabilitate perpetrators.

Substance use. Approximately 15% of the population will abuse substances at some point during their lives. Such substance abuse is associated with a myriad of problems including increased physical (e.g., cardiovascular disease, cancer, liver disease) and mental illness, accidental death, homicide, suicide, and general difficulties in living (job loss, divorce, etc.). The testimony from all spiritual traditions has been a powerful voice in moderating and at times proscribing the use of substances (as in the

Prohibition era). Accordingly, one would expect lower levels of addiction and substance use among spiritually active persons, and, this is exactly what the research shows. Out of 86 studies that examined the relationship between substance use and spiritual involvement, 88% reported a decreased use of alcohol, and 92% reported a decreased use of illicit drugs. For example, in one study of nearly 18,000 college students, those for whom spirituality was very important were three times less likely to use illicit drugs, particularly marijuana, compared to those for whom spirituality was not very important.

Spirituality also may be helpful in the treatment of substance use disorders. For example, Alcoholics Anonymous, which helps individuals to recover from alcoholism, using the 12 steps to recovery, has an average one-year success rate of 34%, somewhat better than other approaches to achieving sobriety. Several of the steps require the member to focus on his/her relationship to God or a Higher Power. For example, in one study, "seeking through prayer and meditation to improve conscious contact with God, praying for knowledge of God's will, and for the power to carry it out," was found to be especially important in sustaining sobriety. Similarly, meditation-based treatment approaches to reduce substance use also emphasize the need to contact God consciously. In a review of 24 studies, all showed positive effects in reducing or preventing substance use. Thus, contact with God through prayer and meditation may be a particularly powerful approach to recovery from drug and alcohol abuse.

Psychopathology. At any one point in time as many as 25% of the population is suffering from a mental illness, and nearly 50% will suffer from some form of mental illness during their lifetimes. Does spirituality decrease one's chances of having a mental illness?

Depression is often called the common cold of mental illness, because it affects so many people. Studies of the relationship between spirituality and depression have examined two broad questions: do high levels of current spiritual involvement *prevent* disease and can spiritually-based interventions help to *alleviate* already developed depression. Of the more than 100 studies of depression and spirituality, greater involvement was found to be associated both with less current (65% of studies) and future depression (68% of studies), and spiritually-based interventions were found to be helpful in the treatment of depression (63% of studies). Moreover, the approximately 1/3rd of the studies that found negative or mixed effects, seemed to result in part by differences in how individuals approached spirituality. That is, some types of spiritual involvement tended to lead to more, not less depression. Individuals who tended to blame God, who avoided problems by immersing themselves in spiritual activities, or who approached spirituality for its external rewards, (e.g., business/social contacts) rather than for an interior connection to God, had higher levels of depressive symptoms. Thus, although spirituality can help both to prevent and treat depression, those who approach spirituality as a way to seek an interior connection to God tend to be more likely to show a benefit.

Mental illness and suicide are often linked; as many as 90% of individuals who commit suicide are suffering from some form of mental illness. In 2008, suicide was the tenth largest leading cause of death, accounting for around 1.5% of all deaths. Most spiritual traditions condemn suicide. Consistent with these prohibitions, out of 68 studies of the association between spiritual involvement and suicide, 84% reported fewer suicides and more negative attitudes toward suicide among spiritual individuals. Tellingly, none of the studies found higher suicide rates among persons with greater spiritual commitment. Thus, there is very clear evidence that spiritual involvement leads to more negative attitudes toward suicide and fewer suicides.

Anxiety disorders range from simple irrational fears, called phobias, to complex and often debilitating illness, such as severe obsessive compulsive disorder, or panic disorder. Most of the studies in this area have examined "neuroses"—a tendency to become worried and preoccupied with concerns. However, the quality of the studies is quite variable. The most reliable studies examined the future development of anxiety among currently healthy individuals and the effect of spiritual interventions in alleviating anxiety among the already afflicted. These studies provide strong evidence that spiritual involvement is associated with less anxiety, with over 80% supporting the positive effect of spirituality on reducing anxiety. For example, studies have shown that both Christian devotional meditation, consisting of prayer, Bible reading and contemplation of biblical material, and formal Buddhist mindfulness meditation can significantly reduce anxiety and panic symptoms in individuals suffering from an anxiety disorder. In addition, similar to the findings with depression, there also is evidence that individuals who turn to spirituality for external reasons of social status or social connection are more likely to be anxious, whereas those who turn to spirituality for the interior connection to God tend to be less anxious. Thus, there is evidence that spirituality may be helpful both to prevent and treat anxiety.

Psychotic disorders are the most severe form of mental illness. Persons affected with psychotic disorders often suffer lifetime illness that can seriously compromise their ability to work, to have a family, and to be independent. In the past, there has been widespread belief among clinicians that persons with psychosis, especially schizophrenia, were preoccupied with spiritual concerns. Thus, the strong expectation was that spiritual involvement would tend to "feed" and exacerbate any underlying psychosis. This concern now seems largely groundless. In fact, persons with schizophrenia appear to be no more preoccupied with spirituality than those who are not mentally ill, and tend to show lower, not higher, levels of spiritual involvement. In addition, of the few studies that have examined the question, most find that spirituality either is unrelated to or decreases the likelihood of psychosis, with only one study reporting that spiritual involvement led to more psychosis. For example, persons admitted for treatment for schizophrenia were less likely to be rehospitalized if they said prayers at least daily, if their families encouraged them to continue to attend spiritual services when in the hospital, or if they expressed an affiliation with a spiritual tradition. Thus, on balance, rather than increasing psychosis, spiritual involvement seems to be more likely to reduce the likelihood of psychosis and psychotic symptoms.

Explanations for the Association between Spirituality and Better Mental Health

There is clear evidence that spiritual involvement leads to increased positive mental health (sense of well being, happiness, marital satisfaction) and decreased mental illness. What is less clear is why. Few studies have explicitly examined potential underlying factors that might explain the association between spirituality and mental health, and of those, most have been limited to examining psychological, social, and physiological explanations as opposed to spiritual ones (God's grace). Nonetheless, several explanations have been suggested and many of them have some empirical support.

Many spiritual traditions promote a healthy personal lifestyle that both encourages healthy behavior (vegetarian diet, hygiene, bodily fitness—Yoga) and discourages risky behavior (alcohol overuse, overeating/gluttony, and sexual promiscuity). For example, Sant Mat, the path that I follow, prescribes a vegetarian diet and forbids use of alcohol and illicit drugs. Both increased healthy behaviors and decreased risky behaviors have been related to better mental health (e.g., exercise and decreased alcohol use tend to be associated with lower rates of depression).

Spiritual traditions also tend to promote social integration and support. Spiritual communities are a reliable source of tangible

90

help (food aid, charity, providing child care or transportation) and emotional social support (advice, spiritual counseling, source of fellowship, and friendship) and provide to members a sense of belonging to a larger community. Numerous studies have shown that persons with greater levels of social support and social connectedness have better mental and physical health. Moreover, spiritual organizations also encourage volunteer work to society, and there is evidence that service to others leads to an enhanced sense of well being.

Spirituality provides a sense of meaning and purpose. When life is viewed as senseless, everyday events can be more difficult to endure, leading to a variety of stress reactions. Spirituality provides a world view that can provide a context for understanding the "slings and arrows" of fate, allowing people to place events in a larger and more intelligible perspective. Spiritual beliefs give people a sense of coherence, an ability to make sense of their lives, rather than believing that they are victims of a random and uncaring universe. Importantly, a sense of coherence and meaning has been related in many studies to better mental health and to lower levels of stress.

Spirituality also may give people a sense of worth, self-esteem, and control. For instance, spiritual traditions often teach that all people are God's children and are loved and valued by God. In addition, most spiritual traditions teach that God is all-powerful and that all things are possible with God. Aligning with a powerful other, like God, may give individuals a sense of vicarious control. There is also modest evidence that spiritual involvement is related to higher self-esteem. Moreover, a sense of control and self-esteem has been consistently related to reduced mental illness.

Spirituality tends to give people a sense of peace, stability and positive emotions. For example, spiritual rituals can be comforting during times of difficulty, as when there is sickness or loss, and also provide a predictable and reliable way to celebrate and mark important life milestones, such as birth, initiation into adulthood, marriage, and death. Spiritual teachings also promise God's help and comfort. This may invoke a sense of optimism and expectancy of positive change that might operate similarly to the placebo effect. Moreover, connecting techniques, such as prayer and meditation have been shown to produce a sense of well being and peace.

Although all of the above are plausible explanations for the helpfulness of spirituality in promoting and maintaining better mental health, to the spiritual person, all fall short. That is, none seriously considers the central tenet of spiritual belief, the immanence or presence of God/Higher power, and God's grace in the world and in the lives of God's followers. To the spiritual believer, any explanation of the association between spirituality and better mental health is incomplete without the inclusion of the notion that God actively intervenes in the lives of humankind for their benefit. Instead, spirituality teaches that God "heals all of our diseases." That is, God is active in the world; God answers prayers and heals the afflicted. Science typically restricts itself to material explanations. Recently, however, science has begun to provide evidence for the effectiveness of spiritual healing. In one recent review of the evidence by Dr. Daniel Benor, roughly two-thirds of over 190 controlled experiments examined showed a statistically significant positive effect of spiritual healing on living beings, including plants, animals, and humans. That is, roughly *thirteen times* more studies were significant than the 5% that would be expected if the results were simply due to lucky accidents or random factors. Thus, both spirituality and science provide reasons to believe in the active intervention of God/Spirit in helping to maintain and promote mental health. Clearly, there is much more work to be done to understand the relationship between spirituality and mental health. However, any complete understanding will need to consider both material (physiology, psychology, social factors) *and* spiritual explanations.

What It Means for Our Lives

There are several lessons that derive from our study of the association between spirituality and mental health. First, the strongest factor associated with better mental health is consistent attendance at spiritual services. That is, although spiritual beliefs or feelings have at times been associated with mental health, active practice of one's spirituality, especially regular attendance at spiritual services or meetings, is related much more strongly. Thus, one lesson is that spiritual belief, without action and application in one's life, is not very effective. For example, Science of Spirituality, recommends regular attendance at "satsang," i.e., spiritual discourse and group meditation, as well as daily meditation practice.

Another important finding is that comparisons between different spiritual traditions, with few exceptions, rarely show differences in mental health outcomes. Those who are spiritually involved tend to have better mental health than those who are not involved, regardless of the specific spiritual tradition or practice followed. Thus, a second lesson appears to be that it is not what spiritual tradition you align yourself with that matters, but how deeply and consistently you follow it. In this regard, the teachers of Science of Spirituality note that there is no need to change our religions; rather, we need to become true followers of our religions.

A third finding was that persons who follow a spiritual path for external reasons, such as social connections in the community, may actually show negative effects of spirituality. In contrast, persons who follow a spiritual path for internal reasons, of connectedness and closeness to God, show positive effects of spirituality on their mental health. Thus, another lesson is that spirituality should be practiced not for its external rewards but for its ability to change us, to help us to form an inner connection to God. As noted by the teachers of Science of Spirituality, the purpose of religion is not to get more things or to achieve a more comfortable life; it is to attain self-realization and God-realization.

A related lesson is that certain practices, especially those that attempt to produce an interior and contemplative closeness to God, such as meditation, may be particularly effective in promoting mental health. Moreover, meditation not only promotes mental health, but also reduces mental illness in those that are currently mentally ill. Thus, the development of a meditative practice might be recommended both as a preventive and as a healing intervention. Sant Rajinder Singh Ji Maharaj, the current Master of meditation on inner light and sound, talks about meditation as being receptive and open to God. In this regard, it is important to note that meditative practices typically require the help of a teacher. In my own life, I was both astonished and transported by the profound difference in my inner experience of meditation following initiation by my spiritual Master, Sant Darshan Singh Ji Maharaj, and the ongoing meditation guidance and help from the current spiritual Master, Sant Rajinder Singh Ji Maharaj.

Closing Thoughts

Mental illness is a potentially debilitating disease, with profound negative effects for the sufferer on their families and personal lives. Psychologists and psychiatrists have labored diligently for more than 100 years to find the causes and effective treatments of mental illness and to identify factors that promote mental health and happiness. In their long search for helpful treatments, mental health professionals have often looked askance at spirituality, seeing it as causing more harm than good. It is ironic that recently spirituality has emerged as an effective and nearly universally applicable intervention to prevent and treat mental illness.

As a psychologist and as a spiritual person, I have been frustrated by the distrust and miscommunication that have at times plagued the on again, off again relationship between spirituality and science. I have been inspired that scientific knowledge and spiritual practice can be reconciled by the examples of my teachers, Sant Darshan Singh Ji, and Sant Rajinder Singh Ji, a spiritual Master who is also a trained scientist. Moreover, in my many years as a teacher and professional clinical psychologist, I have been struck by the dramatic and salutary influence of spirituality in bettering the lives of my students and clients. Spiritual belief and practice bring hope when all else fails. It is my hope that this chapter helps to bridge the divide between these oftentimes disparate perspectives, illustrating the synergistic effects that may occur when both science and spirituality are applied seriously to the problem of mental health. As Sant Rajinder Singh Ji has noted, "Both science and spirituality come to the same truth, but arrive there differently."

John McGrew, Ph.D. earned his Ph.D. in Clinical Psychology from Indiana University. Currently, he is Professor of Psychology and Director of Training for the Clinical Psychology Program at Indiana University–Purdue University Indianapolis, where he serves as an administrator, an educator, and a researcher. His research focuses on evidence-based practices to support and treat two different populations of persons with mental illness: those with severe mental illness and those with autism. His work has been supported by more than fifteen grants and contracts from federal, state, and local agencies and foundations. Dr. McGrew is co-editor of a book on psychological practice in a changing health care system and co-author of a book to be published in 2012 on a new consulting model to enhance educational outcomes for children with autism. In addition, he has published over 60 articles in books or professional journals and made more than 75 presentations at national and regional conferences.

CHAPTER 8

FAQs ON MENTAL HEALTH AND SPIRITUALITY

by Marshall O. Zaslove, M.D.

One out of five people in the United States has a mental illness, and many more millions in their families and communities are impacted by these disorders.[1] Since mental illness is so widespread, and since for forty years I have been a practicing psychiatrist and also a student of the Science of Spirituality, people have frequently asked me questions about the relationship between psychiatry and spirituality.

To help in answering these questions, it was my good fortune to be present at many discussions on the spiritual aspects of medicine and psychiatry with the spiritual Master Sant Darshan Singh Ji Maharaj over the fourteen years of his mission. Sant Darshan Singh Ji took a personal interest in helping to solve the problems people brought to him, and he had a broad and deep knowledge of medical subjects and psychology and their role in the life of the spiritual seeker. These discussions, sometimes at patients' bedsides, sometimes in cars or airports, and sometimes spanning several hours, represent for me the most accurate, insightful, and hopeful body of information on spirituality and psychiatry.

What follows is an attempt to live up to this sacred trust, by passing on as well as I am able some of the wisdom that he left in our care, in the spirit of loving helpfulness for the ill and anguished which he tirelessly exemplified.

Similarly, during the past twenty-three years, Sant Rajinder Singh Ji Maharaj has answered questions and given talks on stress, depression, substance abuse, etc. I will try to summarize this information or indicate where it can be accessed.

The following are some of the questions that spiritual seekers, students of the Science of Spirituality, my patients and their families and friends, and practitioners and caregivers have asked about psychiatry and spirituality. In all cases, I have preserved the questioner's anonymity while giving answers that the interested reader may find helpful.

DISCLAIMER: The following is for information only. If the reader is suffering from a diagnosable mental illness, he or she should seek professional help; do not use what follows as a prescription for individual treatment or management.

Seeking Treatment

[Psychiatrists have not had a reputation for receptivity to spirituality, perhaps because 65% of psychiatrists report having no training at all in spiritual subjects.[2] As a result, many spiritual students have asked whether they should undergo psychiatric treatment, and what they might experience if they do so.]

Question: I am a person with spiritual leanings; should I seek psychiatric treatment for my mental symptoms, or leave it all to God to cure me?

Dr. Zaslove: The short answer: "Yes," if you need it, seek professional treatment; and "No," we should ordinarily not "leave it all to God."

Research shows that even normal thinking processes are prone to error and misunderstandings. Distorted perceptions and confused thinking and judgment are common symptoms of mental and emotional illness. A person with mental illness may not even realize he or she has such an illness.

If you or a loved one suffer from serious mental symptoms, it would be best to arrange for evaluation by a competent professional. Recent research indicates that early treatment of mental illness may prevent advance to more serious conditions. Prompt action can be lifesaving: for instance, depressive disorder and psychosis are each associated with elevated death rates from suicide (one out of ten, compared with one suicide per 100,000 for the general population).[3]

Also, many seemingly "mental" symptoms may actually be caused by medical conditions such as thyroid disease, nutritional deficiency, head injury, drug side effects, stroke, substance abuse or withdrawal, heart disease, infection, etc.—and so can be treated effectively if accurate diagnosis is made by a professional.

Question: How do I know if my mental symptoms are serious enough for me to see a psychiatrist, as opposed to waiting it out and just meditating and doing the spiritual diary [a daily record of ethical living and meditation practices] and hoping for improvement?

Dr. Zaslove: Life has its ups and downs, and a certain amount of stress, sadness, anxiety, etc. is the common lot of every person. Our spiritual Masters tell us that these painful emotions do lessen, if we continue accurate daily meditation under the guidance of an adept, and pursue the ideal of an ethical life (which for students of this science, includes the daily spiritual diary). Gradually, we become less affected by the physical world and its inevitable pressures, wounds, and disappointments.

Major life changes can trigger more distressing symptoms, such as grief and withdrawal after the death of a loved one or a divorce; these symptoms tend to be self-limited and often can be handled by our own efforts, e.g. the use of certain simple homeopathic remedies. If self-treatment does not suffice, crisis counseling from a professional or even from a reliable friend can help.

However, if mental symptoms persist and also interfere with our ability to work or study or maintain relationships for a significant period of time, then evaluation and treatment are needed. Also, if we are too anxious, depressed, excited, or distraught to meditate, then treatment can help us regain our footing on the spiritual path. If our inner turmoil is preventing us from meditating and thereby transcending our problems, then treatment—that may include prescribed medication—can help us regain our equipoise.

Finally, anyone having suicidal or homicidal thoughts, or who is unable to sleep or eat to the point of physical damage, should not delay; *get professional help immediately*.

Question: But won't psychiatric treatment interfere with my spiritual progress?

Dr. Zaslove: No, quite the contrary; untreated mental illness will hinder our spiritual progress. To move forward and be successful in any major enterprise, all our faculties need to be working at full strength, and spirituality is no exception.

The spiritual Masters remind us that a certain degree of illness must be played out at the human level, by going through the usual channels of medical evaluation and treatment. We may have karmas to be finished off with our doctors, nurses, and other caregivers; they add that members of the healing professions follow a high calling (as do teachers).

Students of a spiritual Master of Sant Mat may have their illness karmas softened, and accurate daily meditation can dilute newly-acquired karmas. However, as a general rule, if the karmic debt must be paid off here to prevent our having to come again into the physical form, then we may experience illness.

Spirituality is a path of hope, and hope is an antidote to depression and anxiety. Even when faced with the most serious mental illness, in my personal experience there is never reason to lose hope. Help is available, both within and without, and mental symptoms can be treated, managed, controlled, and often healed. There is never any reason to avoid getting help because of discouragement or hopelessness. I have seen many patients with very serious psychiatric diagnoses regain their health over time, especially those who meditate daily and keep the spiritual diary prescribed by this science.

Sincere prayer is a major part of our lives, but our teachers recommend prayer plus effort as more effective than prayer alone. They explain that, while the Lord's grace is always forthcoming, our own efforts bring forth even more grace, which inspires us to more effort, etc., in a virtuous cycle. This principle holds not only for healing, but also for all our endeavors.

Making the effort to seek help and go through the treatment process is a sound decision from both the worldly and spiritual perspectives.

Question: But what if the psychiatrist says I need to take medications? Won't these drugs interfere with my meditations?

Dr. Zaslove: In my clinical experience, the modern pharmacologic treatments for mental and emotional symptoms do not seem to interfere as much with meditation and other spiritual practices. If carefully prescribed only when indicated, and in appropriate dosages, they are also more effective than treatments were in the past.

I personally helped many of my patients who were taking psychiatric medication to learn to meditate, and often they had very good concentration and meditation experiences while on their medication.

Psychiatrists and Spiritual Seekers

Question: Several years ago I went to a psychiatrist, but I was turned off by his intolerant attitude towards my spiritual practices. He said I was retreating from the real world. Is this a common experience?

Dr. Zaslove: Yes, I think so, because many spiritual aspirants have expressed similar complaints about psychiatrists and other psychotherapists. It is true that in the past, many psychiatrists thought that spiritual and religious practices in their patients were more likely to be irrelevant or even problematic—rather than positive, helpful influences in psychiatric treatment.

Not fully recognizing the positive value of spirituality has definitely been a failing in psychiatry (and in medicine in general), perhaps because of lack of training. Prior to 1994, only three medical schools in this country taught courses on spiritual or religious issues.[4]

Fortunately, this has changed. Psychiatry can no longer ignore the increasing numbers of studies suggesting that spirituality can positively affect mental health.[5]

Question: So are psychiatrists trained to be more tolerant now?

Dr. Zaslove: Since 1995, psychiatric training programs in the United States are required to address spirituality and religion in their coursework, and the American Psychiatric Association's practice guidelines now call for "clinically respectful evaluation" of the spiritual and religious beliefs of every patient evaluated.[6]

Have training and official recommendations helped psychiatrists be more understanding of their patients' spiritual needs and preferences? On a survey, more than half of psychiatrists said spirituality was "very important," and that they would recommend a "spiritual intervention such as meditation" for their patients, if it were found helpful. Discussions are appearing in psychiatric journals about such subjects as how clinicians can distinguish clinical depression from the spiritual seeker's "dark night of the soul" (an uncomfortable period during which both outer satisfactions and inner spiritual experiences are not forthcoming).

Of course, training programs, responses to surveys, and articles in psychiatric journals cannot predict what you will actually encounter when you consult a psychiatrist.

Question: So how can I find a psychiatrist/psychotherapist who will understand the importance to me of my spiritual practices?

[In my experience, this is the single most frequently asked question about spirituality and psychiatry.]

Dr. Zaslove: First, it is usually true that "good people know other good people," so you might ask a friend or professional who has spiritual leanings, whom he or she would recommend as a professional who shares your interest in spirituality.

Another course of action would be to search online the growing body of psychiatric literature on the importance of spirituality in treatment, and contact one of the authors for a referral in your area. There are some organizations of professionals who are interested in spirituality, and their websites might be helpful. Since residency programs now require orientation to patients' spiritual needs, a more recently trained practitioner might be more receptive. Also, people have mentioned to me that doctors from traditional cultures where religion and spirituality are an accepted part of daily life are sometimes more likely to be in tune with one's spiritual aspirations.

Interviewing a professional briefly over the phone before you make an appointment is a generally-accepted practice. You could mention that you are a student of spirituality, and then judge for yourself from the doctor's response to this information whether you can work with him or her.

Talking to Psychiatrists

Question: What is the best way to tell my psychiatrist/ psychotherapist about my search for God so that he or she will understand?

Dr. Zaslove: Common sense would suggest you not blurt out to your psychiatrist at the first visit, "You need to know that my whole life is totally devoted to seeking my spiritual goals, no matter what. I put my inner work ahead of my family, my job, even my health. And don't try to change this." Keep in mind that your psychiatrist will be looking for extremes in thoughts and actions that tend to characterize certain mental disorders.

In fact, Sant Darshan Singh Ji and Sant Rajinder Singh Ji have taken pains to remind us that this is a science of *positive* mysticism, which means *balancing* our spiritual work and our obligations to family, community, and society. If we look at the lives of the spiritual Masters of this science, we see that they cheerfully and lovingly discharged all of their family and social obligations, worked hard and successfully at their careers—and yet also achieved their spiritual goal.

If you inform your psychiatrist that realizing your spiritual aspirations is very important to you, but that you are seeking balance in all areas of your life, you will probably get a better response.

Also, psychiatrists are medically-trained scientists, dedicated to the scientific method. Explaining to your doctor that you are in fact practicing spirituality as a science in which you are testing the hypotheses of spirituality yourself and not just going on blind belief may also reassure him or her. You might add that your spiritual practices, especially regular meditation, support you and help you to maintain moderation and objectivity in your life and are not disruptive. You could remind your physician of the voluminous research showing that the practice of meditation helps reduce stress, depression, anxiety, addictive behavior, etc.[7] Increasingly, practitioners are aware of this information.

Meditation and Common Mental Disorders

Question: I am plagued by phobias, and medications have not helped much so far. Will meditation help?

Dr. Zaslove: Yes, meditation can help; I have seen this myself. A woman came to the lectern after a meditation workshop in southern California some years ago and told me the following story:

About two years earlier, she had developed a severe phobia, or fear, of flying in airplanes. She became so frightened before flying that she would have to stop at the airport cocktail lounge and drink herself almost into insensibility in order to be able to board the plane.

She sought treatment for her phobic symptoms with a psychotherapist, with medications, and with yoga and relaxation exercises, but nothing solved the problem completely, she told me.

Finally, she started meditating, using a simple method of concentrating the attention while relaxing the body. By meditating daily, she said, she gradually began to relax both her mental and physical tension, and after a year or so the fear of flying disappeared.

She is an airline flight attendant.

Not only did meditation spare her the misery of a painful mental disorder, it also saved her career.

Question: Is it safe for people with serious mental disorders, such as psychosis, to meditate?

Dr. Zaslove: From my own clinical experience, I believe it is generally safe, but only if the person has proper guidance, and practices a safe method of meditation.

Several dozen of my patients with such major disorders have learned to meditate, and I have meditated with them, and also observed many of them immediately after they meditated, and for a period of time, months or years, after that.

Although a few of these patients may have been unable to focus their attention well enough to meditate, many others were able to

104

do so. I personally have observed no ill effects from meditation in this group of individuals.

However, this statement needs to be qualified: the meditation method we used was in all cases very simple and natural, involving physical relaxation and voluntary focus of the attention, as taught in Sant Mat. No breathing exercises, outer chanting, visualizing, focusing on the kundalini or lower chakras, etc. was employed. Meditations were usually fifteen or twenty minutes in length, and patients understood they could terminate the process at the slightest discomfort.

If we think about it, major mental illness such as psychosis involves losing one's hold on reality. Since meditation, properly practiced, brings us closer and closer to reality, it is actually a help in such conditions.

Question: How exactly does meditation help people with mental disorders? What is the mechanism?

Dr. Zaslove: I believe the mechanism involves several benefits of meditation that are experienced by all practitioners of meditation, but which are particularly helpful in the management of mental disorders. Here are three of those mechanisms:

Meditation relieves stress. All mental disorders are made worse by stress, and meditation is, I believe, the best antidote to stress. Hans Selye, the physician whose 1956 book, *The Stress of Life*, introduced the term into medical use, recognized stress as a part of life.[8] Most stress comes from the mind, and some comes from tension and dysfunction of the physical body. Since in meditation we relax and rest the physical body while simultaneously controlling and re-focusing our mental processes, it naturally relieves stress and anxiety.

Patients with any type of severe mental disorder (especially schizophrenia and mood disorders such as bipolar illness) are particularly vulnerable to the effects of stress and worry. Any changes in their daily routine such as losing sleep, loss or separation from a loved one, or just the frightening nature of their misperceptions, can set off a serious flare-up of their illness that may last a long time.

Regular meditation over a period of months or years seems to re-set the "emotional thermostat" for stress, and gradually the individual becomes more able to withstand the pressures in his or her life. I have known people suffering from severe psychotic illness who added regular meditation over a period of time to their other treatment, and reported that their frightening delusions and hallucinations gradually lost their potency, so they were able to get on with their lives.

Slipping away for an extra meditation sitting or two—however brief—during times of high stress is also a good idea.

Meditation helps us in taming the mind. People with mental disorders often find their mental processes are untrustworthy or out of their control. They may have ideas that are patently false to external logic or keep going around in their mind obsessively; surges of feeling such as fear, anger, depression, and anxiety which seem to come out of nowhere; irresistible urges to hurt themselves, hurt others, or perform rituals such as repetitive hand washing; and so on through the hundreds of pages of psychiatric diagnostic manuals.

Masters of this science of meditation on the inner light and sound tell us that when we learn to meditate, we are learning a powerful method of dealing with our mind. They add that ethical living as taught in science of spirituality also has a calming and balancing effect on the mind.

Meditation supplements other treatments. Sant Rajinder Singh Ji has mentioned that meditation can enhance other treatments for emotional pain and turmoil. When we go within during meditation, we begin to see our lives from a clearer angle of vision and can recognize the roots of our problems. Then, we can pinpoint the areas in which we need to work, and this accelerates problem-solving with a professional psychotherapist or counselor.

Finally, students are given a direct spiritual experience at the time of their initiation into meditation on inner light and sound—a connection that can only be given by a Master of this science. As we continue to meditate and come in contact with that inner current of light and sound at the third or single eye, located between and behind the two eyebrows, this contact serves as an anchor that stabilizes our lives, both worldly and spiritual. Continued regular contact with this current of light and sound within purifies the mind of negative, distressing, and distracting thoughts, and fills our whole being with divine love and bliss that repair and make whole our emotional selves. This current eventually leads us back to our Home, the Source from which we have come, and to which we yearn to return. Such a connection is actually the greatest gift that we can receive from anyone.

Question: But don't so-called "normal" people have the same problem, controlling their mind?

Dr. Zaslove: Yes, all of us definitely do have trouble controlling our mind—even psychiatrists!

In fact, anyone who does not meditate usually cannot control his or her mind easily. We commonly see successful people with highly developed intellects, or very advanced in the arts, athletics, the professions, or in the financial or political world, subject to sudden impulses, explosive outbursts or mood swings, self-defeating behaviors and addictions, and other wiles of the mind.

This aspect of meditation is important for all of us. Meditation when understood from this point of view has some of the aspects of a panacea, since it helps with so many different physical and mental symptoms, and also with normal function.

However, as with any other treatment or medicine, we have to take it to get the benefit; merely knowing that meditation can help us, or even understanding how it may help, is not enough. Regular daily practice is necessary and is recommended by the Masters of this science of meditation.

The effects can be rewarding. I still encounter former patients who come up to me to remind me of how we meditated together ten or even twenty years ago, and how they have never forgotten the experience. Many tell me they are still benefiting from their practice of meditation.

Question: Isn't mental illness karmic in origin? Can a person do much about this kind of karma?

Dr. Zaslove: Spiritual Masters tell us that about seventy-five percent of what occurs in our life is based on karma, or reactions from previous thoughts, words, and deeds, according to the universal law that every action has an equal—and opposite— reaction. This fact can be experienced directly by any student of this science who attains access to higher realms during meditation.

This seventy-five percent would normally include major illnesses that we experience in spite of our best efforts. Of course, we can also incur illness simply by ignoring the strictures of nature and human biology: for instance, if we eat too much fatty food over a long period, raise our lipids and blood pressure, and suffer a stroke.

However, spiritual Masters also tell us that we have free will in the remaining twenty-five percent of our lives. If we choose to do regular daily meditation under the guidance of a Master of this science, there are many beneficial effects that work to lighten the load of our karmas.

During meditation we do not ordinarily have any new thoughts, feelings, or actions, so we are not incurring any new karmas to plague us. When meditating, students of this science also come into contact with a very positive, powerful current within (the inner light and sound), which has a neutralizing effect on the karmas we may have incurred that day—another very important reason to meditate daily! When we are initiated into the Science of Spirituality, our teacher takes over the load of stored karmas that have not yet reached fruition. In some circumstances he may choose to lighten some of the karmic load that we have to bear in this life so that we can pursue our spiritual practices undisturbed.

Psychiatric Medications

Question: If I am taking psychoactive medications and also meditate, how will these two interact? Can I reduce my medications?

Dr. Zaslove: For the sake of safety, it needs to be said very clearly that *starting to meditate regularly does not mean an individual with a psychiatric disorder can stop taking his or her medications, or even reduce the dosage.*

Many people with mental illness object to taking their medications for various reasons, and are anxious to be "drug-free." But reducing or stopping medications is the most frequent cause of relapse in severe mental illness and should never be undertaken without consulting your physician.

However, one of the subtle benefits of meditation is that it helps some medications to be more effective. If an individual takes their medication just before sitting to meditate, the medication can work itself into the system while the body is relaxing deeply and going into a harmonious, healing mode. The effect is particularly noted with subtle medicines such as homeopathic remedies.

Mind, Soul, and Psychiatry

Question: How does psychiatry understand human consciousness, or the soul, and its place in the healing of mental disorders?

Dr. Zaslove: Today, psychiatry seems once more to be swinging back to the view that treatment of mental illness needs to address the patient's deep mental, emotional, and spiritual needs.

Pioneers in this movement have been psychiatrists such as Herbert Benson, who did research at Harvard in a form of meditation which he called The Relaxation Response forty years ago.[9] These days, many psychiatrists meditate, and when I have given meditation workshops to audiences of psychiatrists, the room is usually full. I find that many psychiatrists who may not yet accept the spiritual significance of meditation are nonetheless coming to appreciate the health benefits of this practice.

In 1978, a psychiatrist, Raymond Moody, published *Life after Life*, the first popular book on the near-death experience (NDE), basing it on his own research with 150 patients who had survived clinical death.[10] They described a dark tunnel, a bright light, a loving figure, and a sensation of joy, love, and peace, transcending anything they had previously known. Confounding those who thought this might be a hallucination, they were able to describe actual events going on in other locations, or what instruments lay on top of a cabinet in the operating room.

As psychiatrists on the one hand become increasingly aware of the salutary effects of meditation and other spiritual practices on our patients' mental health, and as more and more psychiatrists themselves begin to practice meditation, and to experience its benefits firsthand, it is to be hoped that long-held prejudices and narrow points of view will give way. Ahead of us will be a more receptive attitude in the profession, leading to more enlightened forms of treatment for the widespread suffering of mental illness.

The psychiatry of the future is likely to acknowledge the centrality of meditation and spirituality in any comprehensive approach to healing mental and emotional disorders. For, as my own spiritual teachers, Sant Kirpal Singh Ji, Sant Darshan Singh Ji, and Sant Rajinder Singh Ji, teach, on the health of the soul depends the health of mind and body both.

Question: You seem to have a strong inclination toward the spiritual; how do you—or any psychiatrist so inclined—keep from unduly influencing your patients?

[This is the second most frequently asked question.]

Dr. Zaslove: APA guidelines specify that psychiatrists are not to proselytize nor otherwise try to impose their personal beliefs on patients. While it is difficult to conceal fully my own personal, spiritual life, I don't ordinarily mention it to patients unless they inquire. I have habitually striven to separate professional

110

practice—in which I am paid to be objective and neutral—from my spiritual life, which is private and subjective.

Along these lines, I once was given the unusual opportunity to visit Sant Darshan Singh Ji at his government office in New Delhi during a workday. Surprisingly, I observed his demeanor at the office to be completely professional; although he was clearly very highly respected and admired by his co-workers, he gave no hint of his role as spiritual guide to tens of thousands of students. His professionalism while at the office, like so much else in his life, has been a model for me to try to live up to.

Question: The practice of psychiatry being what it is, how have you managed to do it for 40 years, and still meditate every day and follow a spiritual Master?

Dr. Zaslove: In fact, it is my belief that I could never have done it if I did *not* meditate; and without the divine blessing of our spiritual Masters, Sant Kirpal Singh Ji, Sant Darshan Singh Ji, and Sant Rajinder Singh Ji, I could do nothing at all.

Marshall Zaslove, M.D. has been a psychiatric physician for 45 years. In addition to clinical practice, he has published original research in major journals and mentored several generations of resident physicians. He is the author of a best-selling book on medical practice, *The Successful Physician*, and has been a keynote speaker at dozens of medical conferences, including the NIH, AMA, and APA. He was elected to two terms as Chief of Staff at California's largest hospital, and was honored with the State of California's Sustained Superior Accomplishment Award. A meditator for forty years, he gives over one hundred seminars and workshops annually on meditation. He is the father of three daughters and lives in California's Napa Valley.

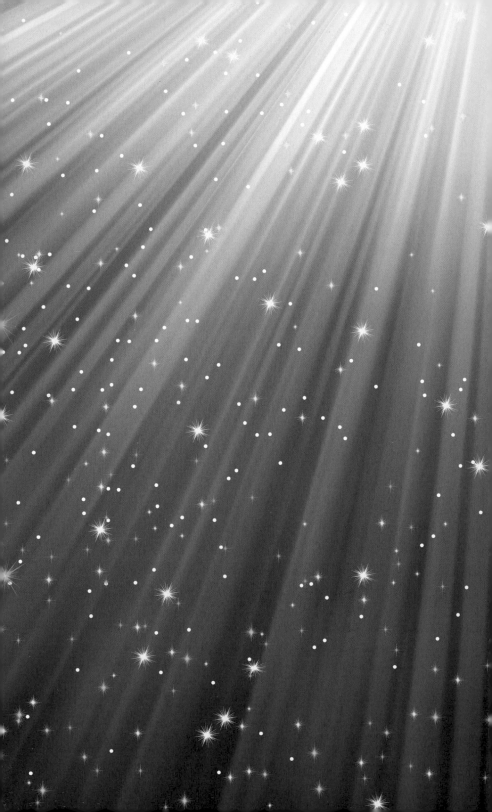

PART 4

Meditation for Balance and Wellness

CHAPTER 9

MEDITATION: FINDING OUR BALANCE

By Rimjhim Duggal Stephens, M.B.B.S.

Amid today's busy lifestyle, I find daily meditation a necessity for my total well-being. Through meditation, taking a moment to calm my thoughts and connect with my soul allows me to withdraw from the world's running pace and return with a sense of peace and serenity. In the modern age, as our involvement in our worldly activities rises, we find our daily personal time dwindles, causing our stress levels to soar and health crises to manifest. While we have recently made tremendous technological strides to seemingly make our lives simpler, we should be cautious that the allure of these advancements does not pull us past the point of productivity and into a realm of physical, mental, emotional, and spiritual imbalance.

As a medical school graduate, I know what it is like to be busy and what it takes to push myself past the daily stressors most doctors experience in their training process. I recall my first clinical rotation focused on surgical training as one of the most demanding specialties—days of waking up at 4 a.m. only to be home late in the evening, yet still having to study before starting again the next day. I would begin the rotation trying to juggle my patients, their histories, clinical exams, lab work, the operating room, and then studying their cases throughout the day and at home. By the third week of this eight-week rotation I felt like I was a hamster on a wheel and would never be able to catch up with all the work I had in front of me. When I first considered meditation, my thought was that if I only had the time I would gladly do it...but where was this time? After another week of this endless schedule, I had had enough and decided no matter what, I would make the time.

I sought out fifteen to twenty minutes to meditate in the morning and within the first few days, noticed that I had more energy as I started my day. I then tried to find times during the day, during lunch, or between surgeries. I was surprised that when I started looking for a few minutes here and there they were actually quite easy to find. Thirty minutes when I woke up, fifteen minutes with lunch, and ten minutes between patients. I was astounded how calm I felt after sitting for even a few minutes, enough that a couple of my fellow medical student colleagues took notice and tried to meditate themselves. Another week passed and I had finally figured it out. Taking out time for meditation did not give me less time; it actually gave me more! I was calmer, more focused, and was able to concentrate better and thus work faster. Although the rest of the rotation was still quite rigorous, my small meditation-breaks provided solace and kept me grounded as I continued the grind. This was luckily an early lesson in my medical career. I have discovered that if we can devote just ten percent of our time to sit in daily meditation, many of life's worries and stressors won't make the impact they once did.

What exactly is meditation? Under the guidance of my revered spiritual teachers, my grandfather, Sant Darshan Singh Ji Maharaj, and my father, Sant Rajinder Singh Ji Maharaj, I have learned that meditation is a process by which we withdraw our attention from the physical senses that connect us to the world around us. This includes withdrawing our sense of sight, touch, taste, smell, and hearing by sitting in silence as we focus on the spiritual connection present within each of ourselves, located in the third or single eye, between and behind the eyebrows. This is achieved through a simple technique called Jyoti Meditation, based on an ancient, time-honored practice known as Surat Shabd Yoga. This scientific method is easy to practice and can be practiced by one of any religion or society. In this method, we close our eyes and learn to look directly in front us, with our eyes in the horizontal plane, focusing about eight to ten inches in front of our forehead. As we quietly concentrate, we feel a sense of calm come over our bodies and mind and we may begin to experience flashes of light or other vistas signifying our connection of our soul with the Divine during our practice. It also helps me to repeat a divine Name of God over and over silently and slowly, so as to still out the thoughts of the world. Over time, we realize that living through only our physical senses limits our vision and that meditation is a method that allows us to tap deeply within ourselves.

Through the use of EEG electrodes, a joint study between Sydney University and the Norwegian University of Science and Technology determined that theta waves were abundant in the frontal and middle parts of the brain during meditation. This indicates that our brain enters a state of deep relaxation that monitors our inner experiences and originates from our collected attention. Alpha waves were also found to be significant in the posterior parts of the brain indicating the difference between concentrated meditative relaxation in comparison to the relaxation experienced while sleeping or resting without applying a specific mental technique.[1] Thus, our brain waves indicate we are concentrated, engaged, and fully conscious while we meditate. To receive the full benefits of meditation, it is important to find a technique that incorporates an inward, relaxed concentration allowing us to experience a connection with our soul.

The benefits of meditation are numerous. Studies of meditators have proved lower blood pressure, increased immune system strength which leads us to decreased susceptibility of illness, and decreased depression, anxiety, insomnia, asthma, fibromyalgia, digestive problems, irritable bowel syndrome, psoriasis, infertility, pain, rheumatologic conditions, and drug or alcohol addiction. Another proven impact of meditation is decreased physical or emotional symptoms associated with chronic illnesses such as heart disease and cancer. One of the most comprehensive studies to be conducted on meditation, The Shamatha Project, led by Saron at the University of California-Davis found that study participants practicing meditation regularly found that their overall sense of psychological function increased, they had greater fluidity in their emotional responses, increased impulse control, improved visual perception, increased focus and attention, and a 30% increase in enzyme (telomerase) activity correlating with major improvements in their sense of purpose in life. Telomerase is an enzyme that is active in living cells protecting genetic material during cell division, and has been found to increase in activity during meditation, suggesting that meditation actually slows our cells from aging in response to stress.[2]

One of the most compelling findings that many physicians agree upon is that people who regularly meditate have a decrease in their variable stress response. We all experience day-to-day stress as we commute, strive to make deadlines, multitask, and deal with our family, friends, health, and homes. When our body perceives threats, our sympathetic nervous system is stimulated and our "fight or flight" system is activated, releasing adrenaline and cortisol that increase our heart rate, breathing, cytokines, and constriction of blood vessels. If this stress response stays "on," the cytokines can produce potentially damaging inflammation throughout the entire body. Meditation is thought to work by reducing activity in the sympathetic nervous system and increasing activity in the parasympathetic nervous system, causing our heart rate and breathing to slow down and our blood vessels to dilate. Not only does regular meditation decrease the body's stress response, but it also provides the body with physical, mental, emotional, and spiritual stability so we don't get "stressed out" in the first place.

As a society, stress-related illnesses have been on the rise in the West and we turn to the East to learn from their centuries of knowledge. Throughout the years, meditation had been thought of primarily as an Eastern tradition, and only recently has the Western world embraced its importance and benefits for both preventative medical care and use as a practical treatment modality. For thousands of years, sages and philosophers in India had left accounts of their meditation experiences and encouraged the process to their students. Throughout the East, the virtues of meditation and the spiritual quest had been ingrained into the ancient cultures and still exists there today. The earliest recorded writings about the meditation process and personal experiences occurred in India about 5,000 years ago in the sacred scriptures known as the Vedas. The sages of those times evolved from performing rituals to elementary stages of meditation, and thence to deeper and deeper states of conscious realization. During the 6th century B.C., Prince Siddhartha looked inward to quiet his mind and seek the secret of happiness for himself and to pass on to his fellow beings. After a reputed forty-nine days of deep meditation, Siddhartha arose with newfound knowledge and became known as the Buddha–the Enlightened One, who over time spread the tradition of meditation from India, to parts of Indonesia, China, and Japan.

Western medicine is now beginning to open its doors to treatment through Ayurveda, acupuncture, homeopathy, and meditation.

Ayurveda and acupuncture are well-established fields that have been practiced for centuries, and have offered effective treatments that are still sought after as natural methods of cure today. Another widely popular system of medicine in the East is homeopathy, which was developed by Samuel Hahnemann (1755–1843) in Germany.

A survey of the medical students at Georgetown University's School of Medicine found that nearly 91% of students thought types of complementary and alternative medicine (CAM) including meditation offered ideas and methods from which Western medicine could benefit. Over 75% of the medical students thought that CAM should be included in their curriculum and felt that knowledge on these types of medicine would be important to them as students and future practicing health professionals.[3]

Ayurveda is a form of medicine that originated in India, detailing numerous natural herbal, medical, and surgical treatments for various ailments that have been found to be quite effective. Nutrition is a big part of this practice and in its own right is a powerful form of preventative medicine.

Acupuncture was developed in China and the underlying principle is that by placing tiny needles in certain points of the body along neural pathways known as "meridians," the flow of energy is restored and illness dissipated.

Homeopathy is a field of plant-based medicine based upon "the law of similars," or "Like cures like." This medical discipline's basic premise is founded on the principle that a substance that causes symptoms of a disease in healthy people will cure that disease in sick people when accurately prescribed by a trained homeopathic physician, in a dynamic yet highly diluted non-material dose of that substance. This has some similarity to the philosophy of vaccination developed in the West, where once given a diluted dose of a material amount of a causative pathogen, one will often prevent a disease from manifesting as an individual builds immunity to that disease. Practitioners in these various fields often prescribe a method of meditation to accompany their recommended treatment modality, and many believe when meditation is used in conjunction, balance is restored more quickly to our natural state.

Meditation has also begun to spread in the field of Western medicine. Due to its vast benefits, a growing number of conventional doctors and healthcare workers are both learning the method of meditation and teaching their patients to meditate. Yearly, there are more medical residencies offering training in preventative medical care, training that often provides teaching doctors how to instruct their patients on meditation techniques to help prevent or delay illness. The combination of meditation with lifestyle and behavior modification is an unparalleled method of illness prevention. One of the top hospitals in the United States, the Mayo Clinic, teaches meditation to patients as part of their Complementary and Integrative Medicine Program. The benefits that meditation can have with illness prevention, concentration, relaxation, inner peace, stress reduction, and fatigue have caused the best medical hospitals and clinics nationwide, such as Stanford and Harvard, to start wellness programs and employ specialists to educate their patients on these positive effects.

Doctors themselves can benefit from practicing meditation. In a recent examination of literature it was found that 28-45% of medical students and 27-75% of resident physicians (depending on their specialty) as well as numerous practicing physicians undergo a state of "burnout" at least once in their career. Burnout is a state of repetitive stress causing mental and physical exhaustion related to work or care-giving activities. Burnout during residency training has received significant attention as concerns regarding patient care and job performance are on the line. Time demands, lack of control, work planning, work organization, difficult job situations, and interpersonal relationships are all considered factors in residents' burnout.[4] If doctors are not allowed to take care of themselves and are pressured to the point of burnout, how can we expect them to also take on responsibility for their patients' lives?

A twenty-two month study from the Southern Illinois University School of Medicine's Medical/Dental Education Preparatory Program found that students who participated in their meditation exercises regularly in two classes had decreased test anxiety, nervousness, self-doubt, and concentration loss. They felt that meditation activity helped them academically and would help them as a physician.[5] Burnout is not limited to physicians but can occur in anyone with a stressful life situation and in any line of work. Workplace interventions have begun to be put in place across all fields. Workload modifications, diversity of duties, stress management training and wellness workshops are among the top methods of education offered.

With many patients, I have noticed that the combination of meditation, dietary and social habit changes, along with exercise, has helped them with a range of their current illnesses as well as reducing their risk factors for future diseases. Preventative medicine is gaining more popularity as a field and is the most affordable method of health care we have. Meditation is free. All we need to do is to sit in silence and withdraw from our physical senses. It can be done anytime during the day at home, at work, at school, in a park, or even in our car. Eliminating mind-altering substances such as alcohol and drugs offers us a cost savings as well as major health benefits. Reducing the consumption of animal foods, or eliminating them altogether, while adopting more fresh plant-based foods, preferably organically grown, may seem more expensive in the short term but is definitely much less expensive if we can avoid hypertension, diabetes, and pesticide exposure in the future. Exercise can also be practiced without a cost. We can do many forms of exercise without even heading to a gym. With the variety of video classes, online workout sessions, and regular recreational activities, our options are limitless.

In conclusion, the key to living a healthy lifestyle is to recognize the need for balance and then strive to achieve it. We are living lives where we are sometimes pulled to take care of the physical, emotional, or mental part of us and we often focus on one at the expense of the others. By regularly meditating, we will gain insight on how to connect to the spiritual part of our being, which is the most often forgotten. Once given some attention, this spiritual part will help guide us to achieve the balance we are looking for. It starts with a simple step: sitting down, closing our eyes, and allowing ourselves to feel a spiritual connection. Once we have experienced ourselves as soul we will lead healthier, happier lives filled with purpose, serenity, and balance. As we each find inner contentment, we will be able to pass it onto our family, friends, colleagues, and neighbors allowing meditation to peacefully transform the world through our united connection with the Divine.

Rimjhim Duggal Stephens, M.B.B.S. began pursuing her medical degree at the prestigious Manipal University in southern India. There she learned her core basic sciences and developed an interest in alternative medicine. She then focused on her clinical sciences at The University of the West Indies where she gave the valedictory address upon receiving her medical degree. Dr. Duggal Stephens now resides in Vancouver, Canada, where she is focusing her attention on wellness through the nutrition and homeopathic sciences as well as continuing her meditative practice. She has studied meditation under the guidance of Sant Darshan Singh Ji Maharaj and Sant Rajinder Singh Ji Maharaj for over twenty years and lectures on the benefits of meditation, optimum health through the vegetarian diet, and wellness through preventative medicine. Dr. Duggal Stephens has researched numerous healthcare modalities available around the world and has chosen to focus on a preventative and integrative approach to medicine.

CHAPTER 10

MEDITATION AND SPIRITUALITY: A HOMEOPATH'S PERSPECTIVE

by Timothy W. Fior, M.D., D.Ht.

Spirituality in general and meditation in particular can influence our physical, mental, emotional, and spiritual health. I have found over the last twenty-four years of practicing conventional medicine and homeopathy[1] that spirituality and meditation can have an impact on both physician and patient alike. When I sit for my meditation practice every morning, I find that it recharges me for another day at the office while seeing patients. When I have done sufficient and proper meditations, I find the day flows by easily and any problems seem to skim right off my back without disturbing me. However, if I cut corners on meditation, I find simple encounters become difficult. A physician colleague has even found that doing a meditation practice in which we focus on inner light while repeating God's name (called the *simran* practice) can be life saving. While he was in training at a very busy public hospital, he found that he was often called upon to treat very sick and dying patients. He was often overwhelmed at the task. As he had just been initiated, he resorted to simran while around these patients and amazingly found that they often stabilized and improved. He became so well known for his ability to stabilize desperately ill patients that nurses would often pull him from room to room in the emergency department. However, the personal benefits of meditation are not limited to initiates. My father-in-law who is not initiated has found that even 10-15 minutes of meditation once or twice a day will help problems that are not relieved by any medicine. All this occurs without side effects to which he is quite prone.

To understand the health benefits of meditation and spirituality, we can begin by describing what health is. Health is a state of balance of body, mind, emotions, and spirit according to both homeopathic philosophy and the WHO.[2] Disease, according to homeopathy, is an imbalance in any one or combination of these levels. Homeopathic medicine is holistic in that it combines body, mind, and emotions in both diagnosis and treatment. However, Samuel Hahnemann, the founder of homeopathy, recognized the importance of spirituality and God in health. Sant Darshan Singh Ji Maharaj used to quote Hahnemann as saying, "The doctor prescribes, but it is God that heals." This is an aspect of medicine that many physicians, patients, and family members forget. Sometimes, despite all efforts at restoring health, no progress is made. Then, in another situation that is seemingly similar and the prognosis is grave, the patient makes an incredible recovery that amazes everyone including the physician. Encountering situations like this on a regular basis, we are forced to either become disheartened or to do our best and leave the rest to God. The first approach can lead to sadness and even disease, whereas the second approach allows us to maintain our equipoise in life and prevents compassion fatigue. This second approach allows us to be passionate about the treatment but dispassionate or detached from the outcome.

Scientific evidence that meditation helps us to achieve some state of balance is found in some recent EEG coherence experiments. An EEG or electroencephalogram is a recording of the electrical activity of the brain usually taken from a series of electrodes placed on the scalp. For the average awake person, the correlation or coherence of electrical activity between the left and right brain is minimal (less than 10% coherence). When the subject meditates, the EEG patterns of the left and right brain begin to synchronize more and more. For an experienced meditator in a deep state of meditation, the level of synchronization or coherence between the left and right hemispheres can reach an astonishing 99.8%![3] It is truly astounding that while the person is feeling more at peace or in balance during meditation, the EEG recording is also demonstrating exactly that—a balancing between the two sides of the brain. This phenomenon also has a transpersonal aspect. Not only do the two sides of the brain of a single subject become coherent during deep meditation, but also the left and right brains of different people meditating together also manifest nearly identical patterns. Experiments with groups of up to 12 people meditating together have show brain synchronization rates over 80%.[4] This may also serve as objective evidence of the altered states that people report while in India and meditating in groups of thousands of people. This alteration of brain wave patterns between hemispheres is not unique to meditation, as it has also been found to occur in individual patients having an exceptional response to homeopathic remedies.[5] In one study, exceptional responders exhibited significant changes in prefrontal EEG cordance. This is an indication of increased blood flow in the prefrontal cortex, which is known to control executive function and attention. Thus, both the process of meditation and responding to a homeopathic medicine create demonstrable effects on the functioning of the brain.

If we include spiritual health in our overall definition of health as suggested above, the relative importance of meditation and prayer becomes obvious. These are the two main ways of attaining spiritual balance in our lives. Prayer is common to the exoteric forms of all religions. It consists of talking to God, usually to ask for help in some area of our lives. Meditation is the quieting of the mind so that we can hear God's response.

It is common to the esoteric form of all religions. Of the two, it has been my experience that meditation is the superior form. Although prayer is more active in that we are beseeching God for something, meditation is an attempt to still the body and the mind. In life, value is generally put on doing things, thus the value of trying to do seemingly nothing as in meditation is difficult to understand. However, those who meditate successfully can readily feel the benefits.

One way to understand the importance of meditation is to try to look at things from God's perspective. God listens to prayers all the time, but people can only hear responses if they are in a meditative state and have quieted their minds. Thus, meditation is the only opportunity for God to have a true dialogue with us. The importance of dialogue is always obvious in the office. Patients who come in, want to have a monologue and tell what their problem is and how to solve it, and do not respond to suggestions generally do not get better. Conversely, patients who are ready for a dialogue with their practitioner, and who are ready to truly listen to what the practitioner is saying, are much more likely to get better. As Sant Rajinder Singh Ji Maharaj is so fond of saying, how can one fill a glass if it is turned upside-down or it is already full?

In homeopathy, we are aware that people's sensitivity to various environmental factors varies between individuals. In addition, individual susceptibility to various diseases varies from person to person. The emphasis becomes treating an individual who is sick according to his or her own unique sensitivities and susceptibilities rather than treating a particular disease. In homeopathy, each case of disease is unique as is the individual's path to wellness or health. One of the strengths of homeopathic treatment is that it can lessen individuals' chronic susceptibility to various conditions (e.g. recurrent bronchitis or sinusitis). Likewise, in spirituality, we recognize that although God gave us all souls, we are all unique. We are all individuals with free will and differing experiences of life. We are all on a path back to God as well. Sant Rajinder Singh Ji spoke once of how it was God's will that we each be different and unique. It is up to us to rise above our apparent differences to see the unity that resides within. We can do this by calming our mind with meditation.

There are many different systems of medicine in the world just as there are many different types of yogas and meditation. Homeopathy, because it involves highly diluted medicines,[6] is one of the safest forms of medicine. In fact, serious adverse effects from the medicines are virtually unheard of. Herbal medicines are not as safe, and serious adverse reactions have been reported. Conventional medicines, although many were originally derived from plants, are so concentrated and pure that serious even life-threatening adverse reactions are not uncommon.[7] Meditation likewise is a much safer way to a transcendent experience than recreational drugs or near-death experiences (NDEs). Drugs harm the physical body and the mind and do not offer any lasting spiritual gain. I spoke to one long time meditator who used to experiment with hallucinogenic drugs. He felt that his drug-induced experiences were like sneaking into God's house from the back door. He described it as if you are always quite wary and do not feel like you really belong there, as if you have just barged your way in. Conversely, he felt that in meditation he was invited into God's house through the front door. He was welcomed, loved, and felt at home. NDEs likewise by their nature often involve some sort of serious trauma to the body, as the person must be near death to have them. Sant Rajinder Singh Ji says that in NDEs people just approach the threshold of the inner realms. Whereas in meditation, without any physical trauma, we are able to soar into the inner realms all the way back to our true home, the Source from where we came, called Sach Khand (true Region), which is a purely spiritual region. Thus, there are traumatic ways, and there are tranquil ways, such as meditation, to transcend physical consciousness.

There are different ways of categorizing meditation practices. Some meditations concern control over the motor currents and the pranayamas of the body. Because these types of motor current meditations can affect the heart rate and the breathing, they can be dangerous for the very young and the very old. Conversely, meditation on the inner light and sound as taught by Masters of Sant Mat involves withdrawal only of the sensory currents. The motor currents are left alone and the breathing and circulation go on normally. Thus, meditation on inner light and sound is one of the safest forms of meditation. Although it brings many physical, mental, and emotional benefits, as we will discuss later, it is by its nature a purely spiritual type of meditation. The entire emphasis is on the yoking or union of our soul back to God. Any other benefits are merely by-products of this primary aim.

Because meditation on inner light and sound brings spiritual gain to our soul, which is spirit and by its very nature immaterial, the flight of the soul back to God is by its nature not something that can be experienced outwardly in this physical world. To begin this inner journey, time needs to be spent sitting silently and sweetly in meditation. Often, others who are only used to measuring success by outer material gains do not understand the benefits of sitting in silence for spiritual gains. The situation is similar in homeopathy because of the infinitesimally small dose of the medicines given. Until it can be proven how these medicines actually work, some cannot believe that such an infinitesimal dose can work in this material world. However, two hundred years of experience and a fair amount of research reveals that these highly diluted medicines do indeed have an effect.[8] It is truly humbling that despite all the technological advances of our age, we still have not unlocked the mysteries of the soul or of homeopathy. Although this may be troubling to some, it is all a matter of perspective. Regarding our perspective, Sant Rajinder Singh Ji describes how we are more than just a physical body; we are actually a spiritual being or soul that inhabits a body during our physical lifetime that wants to experience the spiritual realms from which it originally came.

Homeopathy can be called the medicine of experience. One cannot learn its art from a book. One can only truly grasp it in the consultation room while seeing patients day in and day out. Because of its seemingly unbelievable tenets, many only come to have faith in it once they have a direct experience of a homeopathic remedy helping something that was not helped by conventional medicine. More converts to homeopathy have been won by the use of the remedy Arnica montana for trauma than probably any other remedy. Masters of Sant Mat likewise teach that the spiritual path is one of experience. It is not one merely of erudition and book learning. We must repeat the experiment ourselves with the instrument of our own being and see for ourselves. Only then can we prove the hypothesis of spiritually for ourselves. There is no place in Sant Mat or in homeopathy for blind belief. Sant Kirpal Singh Ji often said that one is not to just blindly believe what a Master has said but must go within to experience the truth for oneself. He also has said, "What one person has done, another can also do." As we travel on the spiritual path, there are guideposts that help keep us on the path. In homeopathy, likewise there are ways in which symptoms change over time which tell us if we are heading along the path to healing.[9]

Because this is a spiritual path of experience, as we have more experiences, we are empowered more and more on our inner journey. Sant Mat teaches that although the Master is our guide, we can ourselves meet God face to face. Homeopathy is similarly empowering of patients, as most of the medicines are available over the counter and, with experience, the patients are able to treat many problems on their own. The homeopathic physician becomes more of a teacher and a guide, rather than one who must be followed blindly without proving by direct experience the truth of what is being said.

Certain virtues are important on the spiritual path, and one of the most important is that of nonviolence. Gandhi Ji showed the world that the path of nonviolence could defeat an army. Nonviolence in thought, word, and deed is essential to make progress on the spiritual path. Homeopathic medicines are prepared in a nonviolent way in that no animal testing needs to be done. Medicines are first tested in tincture or diluted doses on healthy people and then are used on the sick. Some remedies are made from animal products (e.g. Apis mellifica from the honeybee), but a few specimens can produce remedies for thousands of people because the medicines are so diluted. Hahnemann lived in an era two hundred years ago when the insane were routinely beaten and chained. He pioneered the humane treatment of the mentally ill in medicine. He discouraged any forms of torture and recommended that the insane be treated humanely and gently with homeopathic remedies.

Over the years of homeopathic practice, I have found that many patients benefit from meditation. Those who are open to trying it almost universally say that it helps their mental and physical symptoms. Often, they also achieve some level of spiritual insight as well. I encourage them to do it daily for several weeks in the same place and at the same time so that it becomes a habit. Although at first the mind rebels, after meditating daily for four to six weeks, one feels like something is missing if a day is skipped. It is common for doctors to send patients for a consult to another doctor with more expertise in a certain area. People can likewise get guidance from a spiritual Master who can help enhance their spiritual progress.

Quite a bit of research has been done on how meditation can affect our health. The spiritual benefits of meditation are well laid out in Sant Rajinder Singh Ji's books, such as *Empowering Your Soul through Meditation*, *Inner and Outer Peace through Meditation*, and *Spark of the Divine*.[10] The mental, emotional, and social effects will be covered in other chapters of this book, so I will confine myself to physiological and physical effects of meditation. There are a few caveats that must be given when looking at the research on the effect of meditation on specific health conditions. First, many of these studies are small (i.e. low N or number of participants) and/or single studies that make final or general conclusions impossible. Secondly, certain types of meditation[11] have received most of the research focus. Some researchers have shown that different types of meditation have differing physiologic effects on the body. Therefore, different types of meditation could also affect various illnesses in different individuals in unique ways.

Thirty years ago, researchers began exploring the physiologic effects of meditation on the human body.[12] They found that meditation lowered metabolic rate more rapidly and profoundly than sleep, slowed the brain waves,[13] lowered heart rate and blood pressure and respiratory rates generally, and lowered blood lactate levels. Blood lactate is produced by the anaerobic metabolism of skeletal muscles. Increasing blood levels of lactate are associated with anxiety, and if infused intravenously, can precipitate a panic attack. Because these things indicate a decreased activity of the sympathetic nervous system and represent a hypometabolic, restful state, Herbert Benson called this the Relaxation Response. The opposite hypermetabolic state is the well-known fight or flight response. Research that is more recent has explored the effects meditation has on the hormonal and immune systems. In addition, research has addressed the clinical impact of meditation on particular physical and psychological disorders. Most recently, functional neuroimaging[14] has allowed exploration of the neurophysiological correlates of meditative states, including changes in regional cerebral blood flow and neurotransmitter levels in various parts of the brain.[15] Examples of changes in the levels of neurochemicals in the serum, which are seen during meditation, include increased GABA (an inhibitory neurotransmitter) level[16]; increased melatonin and serotonin levels,[17] and decreased cortisol and norepinephrine levels which are associated with the fight or flight response. Although elegant, all these studies have one glaring deficiency. They do not address the spiritual aspects of meditation. Quite obviously this is true because science has no instrument or other methodology to study the spirit or soul. One reviewer of meditation research poignantly suggests that for research to progress, researchers may need to begin meditating themselves. Only by direct practice and experience of meditation can they remove their blindness to the greater significance of meditation experiences. Perhaps one area of contemporary research that has begun addressing the spiritual issues is the field of near-death experience (NDE) studies.

Researchers have shown that meditation may be an effective intervention for: cardiovascular disease (possibly lowering blood pressure, cholesterol, and risk of heart attack); chronic pain (in fibromyalgia); anxiety and panic disorders; substance abuse; dermatological disorders (like psoriasis); gastrointestinal disorders (like irritable bowel syndrome); respiratory disorders (asthma); neurologic disorders (decreasing seizure frequency in epilepsy); oncological disorders (improves the psychological distress of cancer patients); and reducing medical symptoms in people whether or not they are seeking medical care.[18]

At this point we can ask: Are there any deeper reasons why we meditate and try to attain health? Or what is the true purpose of life? All the goals discussed so far are physical, emotional, or psychological goals. Is there a greater goal? Masters of Sat Mat teach that the ultimate purpose of meditation, spirituality, and indeed life is to achieve self-knowledge and to reunite our soul with God. We achieve self-knowledge when we experience ourselves as soul. To reunite with God, our soul must go on an inner journey through the inner regions guided by the inner light and sound.

One of the first times I become aware of this inner light occurred in college while volunteering to help an elderly woman. Before I met her, she had a cardiac arrest and had a NDE. In that experience, she saw a beautiful, loving, warm light that caused her instantly to lose her fear of death. I could tell by the way that she spoke that she would no longer be afraid to die. The field of near-death studies is a burgeoning one. This area of study suggests that we are not just the body or the mind. People who have NDEs go through several stages, which often culminate in experiencing light, beings of light, and/or a region of light. One researcher looked at adults who as children had experienced an NDE. He found that those who reached the light came back to have their life transformed. They became more loving and caring, took better care of their health, and went more into service-oriented professions.[19]

The year 1988 was a turning point in my own life. I had just finished a family practice residency and was trying to decide in what direction to take my practice of medicine and my life. At the end of the year, I was at Kirpal Ashram in Delhi, India, studying with my spiritual teacher, Sant Darshan Singh Ji Maharaj. This was the last time I was to see him physically and on this encounter he gave me the gift of homeopathy. Although trained in conventional medicine, I was intrigued by homeopathy and wanted to study it more so that I could incorporate it into my practice at some point. Without even asking, he said that I could practice conventional medicine, or a mixture of it with homeopathy or just homeopathy alone. At the time, this guidance seemed puzzling to me as I was not yet a homeopath, but it encouraged me to pursue my study of homeopathy with a newfound zeal. I realized a few years later while talking to Sant Rajinder Singh Ji Maharaj that in fact Sant Darshan Singh Ji Maharaj had laid out for me in this answer my future for the next several years as I transitioned from a conventional medical practice to a mixed practice then to a completely homeopathic practice. Such is the way that spirituality and a spiritual Master influenced my life.

My personal experience with the inner light and sound came in early 1989 while my father was very sick and dying of cancer. He suffered greatly, and on one flight home, I prayed to my spiritual Master to show me a sign that God was watching over my father. I was beginning to question whether the Masters actually do watch over our loved ones as promised. When I arrived at my parents' home, I got to spend time alone with my dad so that my mom could have a break. One day while walking him outside to get some sun, he spontaneously said that he heard some inner music. Instantly I knew that the Master was answering my prayer and that my father was in good hands on his journey back to God. He would be fine even as he passed from this physical world.

In conclusion, I find meditation and spirituality an integral part of life and my medical practice. Meditation makes me more concentrated and attentive to patients as is required in homeopathic practice. In addition, with meditation I have found that it has helped many patients who are looking for ways to deal with many health problems as well as the usual ups and downs of life. The meditation on inner light and sound helps one to evolve spiritually and achieve the true goal of our lives, which is self-knowledge and God-realization.

Timothy W. Fior, M.D., D.Ht. is in private practice at the Center for Integral Health in Lombard, Illinois. For over 20 years, he has practiced Family Medicine and Homeopathy. He is currently a lecturer in the naturopathic program at National University of Health Sciences. He has lectured at many of the medical schools in Chicago and provides clinical rotations for medical students and practicing physicians. He is the current Vice-President, former President, and a founding member of the Illinois Homeopathic Medical Association. He has had many articles published in professional journals and has been quoted in various media on health. He has been a meditator and lactovegetarian for over 25 years.

CHAPTER 11

CHIROPRACTIC AND MEDITATION: FROM HEALING TO WHOLENESS

by Alan R. Post, D.C

Introduction

It has been said that if one had all the wealth and riches of this world, but did not possess health, then they would have nothing of value. Over time, we all come to realize that our health is our greatest asset, for without it, how can we aspire to successfully create, achieve, or accomplish in life? How could we hope to pursue our goals, live our dreams, and explore our vision? It is our body that transports us through this physical world of time, space, and matter, allowing us to be in and experience creation. It is through this life opportunity that we can seek the meaning and purpose of our own creation.

Regardless of whether you have the perspective that you are a physical body having a spiritual experience, or are a spiritual body having a physical experience, it is our structural form that gives us the supportive foundation to move through time and space in this realm of existence. Our structural body provides the framework for the expression of life's movement through the energy of minute subatomic particles organizing into atoms, molecules, cells, organs, and then to ultimately become us: a human being.

137

Our body provides us a coordinated functional organism capable of travel through this magnificent and miraculous world. For those who have lost their health, nothing is more important than seeking its restoration. We have sought health's return through many varied and diverse means since the beginning of our human history.

So too has it been with a loss of one's "spiritual" health. At some point in our life there comes a profound moment of spiritual awareness. We need the answers to the universal questions. "Why? Why was I created? What is the meaning and purpose of my life?" Some may only experience it at the time of their transition of passage from this world; others, at the time of loss of a loved one, some life-altering event, or simply in a moment of insight. This realization of a need for answers to life's questions can initiate in us a profound transformation when it does occur. How can we connect to truth—that eternal essence that is at the core of our being and that of all creation? How can we again become at one, unified with that pure, scintillating, pulsating energy of life that animates all living forms in the cosmos?

I know that chiropractic physicians can play an important role in facilitating the reclaiming of our physical health when it has been lost. As well, they can provide valuable benefit in the maintenance of our health throughout life. Sometimes the line and boundary that differentiates the physical from the spiritual is not so easily delineated. Having been blessed with the opportunity to serve through practicing the chiropractic science and healing art since 1982, and having treated thousands of patients, performed hundreds of thousands of chiropractic specific procedures, I can address this subject. With my pursuit of answers to life's questions leading me to initiation into meditation practices back in 1977, I can speak from personal experience about one's spiritual quest as well. There is a miraculous and fantastic opportunity available to all of us for the achievement of our goals for physical and spiritual health through the utilization of chiropractic health care and meditation. Let us explore these realms of art and science to understand how both can take us on the path toward health and wholeness!

Chiropractic and Health

In the 19th century, there was a renaissance in the healing arts and sciences in the Western world. With the advancement of new inventions, techniques, and procedures — from anesthesia to public health and hygiene, and the incredible new ability to see inside the body with the discovery of x-rays, our understanding of how the body functioned and how we could affect health was revolutionized. It was toward the later portion of the 19th century that a Canadian living in America, Dr. Daniel David Palmer, developed a theory as to the cause of the illnesses and infirmities that afflicted humankind. He was a man of diverse interests and studies, which ranged from anatomy to magnetic healing. He postulated on current theories of the time that related to a "Universal Intelligence" that created and organized life in the creation. He went on to theorize that the universal intelligence that created the cosmos interfaced with humans via an "Innate Intelligence" that flowed through the human body systems organizing the miraculous functions that maintain our health and life. He was aware of the body's natural tendency to seek homeostasis and balance, maximizing necessary function in situations as stress or change that affected it. Palmer believed that any interference to an individual's flow of innate intelligence would manifest in an inability of that individual's homeostatic mechanisms to be able to respond and function properly, thereby reducing the ability for health to be expressed. He conceptualized that it was at the level of the spinal vertebrae that the major interference to innate intelligence would most significantly occur. It is at these spinal joints that the spinal nerves interface, entering and exiting the spinal cord for communication with the brain. The nervous system sends and receives messages between the brain and every cell in the body. He termed this disruption of the normal spinal joint function as the "vertebral subluxation." At this location, inhibition, activation, or alteration of nerve messages to and/or from the spinal cord would most likely occur. This impairment to the flow of the nerve messaging disrupts the innate intelligence and hence would disrupt the body's natural homeostatic mechanisms, affecting a loss of health. He further theorized that if the physician could determine where the interference was and remove it utilizing the specific techniques he created, then the flow of the innate intelligence would be released to flow optimal throughout the nervous system: communicating, functioning, and restoring health.

Modern scientists continue to study the subluxation phenomenon. Neuroscientists have known for decades that communication of information travels via the interface of nerve cells. The messages travel from cell to cell via a synapse point between them. There, through chemical, electrical, and vibratory phenomena, the message is conveyed throughout the nervous system. When stress factors exceed the capacity of a joint system to respond normally, a subluxation will occur. Often it is due to a stress-induced event that causes a "buckling" to occur. It can be macro in nature, causing obvious damage to the related tissue and structures in strain and sprain injuries; with the localized symptoms of pain and gross mobility impairment. It can also be micro in nature, causing true functional changes, with little or no obvious damage to related tissue and structure and, with no obvious gross mobility loss or localized symptomatology.

There is an interconnectedness of the body's different systems that seek to insure survival in the unique environments of creation. No system is more critical to us then our nervous system in this process. It takes in information, processes it, and then conveys message responses that allow for dynamic, instantaneous communication and response. The nervous system acts to integrate, coordinate, and communicate the functioning of all other vital systems—hormonal, circulatory, lymphatic, etc.

The role of the chiropractic physician is to remove interference to the body's neurological, biomechanical, and communication pathways, thus enabling them to function optimally. The power that made the body, and which governs the body, ultimately heals the body. A doctor does not heal a patient. It is the patient's own intrinsic homeostatic mechanism that facilitates healing.

Dr. Palmer's treatments restored health to people who were suffering from many diverse conditions. His results were phenomenal! News spread quickly and soon there were great numbers of patients flocking to his clinic in Davenport, Iowa. It was not long before he opened the first chiropractic school to educate, teach, and train other doctors to practice this new healing art. He named it "chiropractic," from the Latin: to be done by hand.

The chiropractic adjustment can both have a local effect of relieving one's pain or discomfort at the site of the subluxation, as well as affecting more complex systemic effects via the nervous system, thus effecting body functions distant from the subluxation area. We are still learning of these mechanisms and how these interactions can stimulate the intrinsic healing response for a patient. In an exemplary study performed in 1991, it was found that white blood cells, our immune system defenders, demonstrate enhanced phagocyte activity (the ability to consume and destroy other cells recognized as foreign and undesired), following chiropractic adjustments to the spine.[1] There is a multitude of research studies, too numerous to reference or review here, that are helping us understand the profound impact that a chiropractic adjustment can have.

Palmer believed that it was the role and responsibility of the chiropractic physician to detect and correct the subluxations, wherever they may be found in the body. This then became the unique core training of the chiropractic physician that differentiated them from all other physicians in the healing arts. As time has passed, and with it the growth and evolution of our knowledge and awareness of science; so too has the training of chiropractic physicians. However, the art of detecting, locating, and correcting spinal subluxations, and any other anatomical areas of disrelationship, buckling, and/or mechanical or neurological interference affecting the health of an individual, still remain central to the chiropractor's approach to healing and wellness. Chiropractic physician training is rigorous, extensive, and comprehensive. It provides the requirements for degree certification and licensing that is recognized in all 50 states and in numerous countries around the world.

When the body and its component parts are not "at ease," a state of "dis-ease" will ensue. This "dis-ease" state can be the origin of one's illness or "disease" process. It is the natural response of the body to seek balance and homeostasis when affected by change or stress. Few are aware that gravitational forces at work in the realm of physics and affecting all matter in the cosmos have a significant effect on our own health. In the seemingly simple act of walking upright, we humans defy some of the universal laws of gravity. Chiropractic physician's structural focus is to remove the negative effects of gravitational forces and eliminate "dis-ease" from the body.

Modern chiropractors have training as well in the science of microbiology and immunology, studying the effects that bacteria and viruses, etc., can all have on the human body. While that effect cannot be ignored, chiropractic has always focused on the resistance of the host. That will best determine the extent that those effects can have on the individual. It is important to be aware that all but the most unusual and virulent of bacteria and viruses surround us all the time. Whenever there has been a plague or epidemic, all are exposed, yet only some succumb. Chiropractic has always been about the creation of a host environment that, through the natural ideal expression of health, will be most resistant to disease.

In the past few decades, research has also revealed the incredible role that our emotions can have on our health and our ability to resist disease. The connecting link to releasing certain chemical neurotransmitters, science has now traced to human feelings. They have a direct effect on the hormonal response of our glandular and immune systems and the ability of our body to fight and/or succumb to disease. Positive emotions such as those of joy, love, and happiness, do indeed affect our physical body and emotional health in very significant ways. Negative emotions like hate, fear, anger, and sadness have other deleterious effects. Studies have demonstrated that even the simple act of smiling has a positive stimulatory affect on our immune system, thus affecting and enhancing our ability to fight off or fall victim to the common cold virus.[2]

With their knowledge, the chiropractic physician can locate and treat many problems that may be interfering and inhibiting our body's natural innate wisdom and tendency toward the expression of optimum health. However, sometimes treatment interventions alone are unable to alter the course of one's condition. There may be other factors affecting health that reside outside the domain of our physician's ability or even our own personal control. These factors could be from our environment, genetics, or emotions, etc. Ultimately, all an individual can do when it comes to health and healthcare decisions is strive to make them impeccably. Having a competent and caring chiropractic physician as an ally in one's quest for health, healing, and wholeness is one of those important decisions.

Healing and the Spirit

The word "healing" comes from the word root sound "ha." It is found in languages from all different regions of the earth: from the ancient Sanskrit language in India, to the ancient

Greek and Latin languages of Europe, to the traditional Native Languages of North and South America. As one researches the common definitions of the word healing, you find it includes: "being whole, hale, vibrant, sound, and light." It is associated with: "attunement, happiness, frequency, consciousness, and wellness." To seek health, one must move from darkness to light, from discord to music, from chaos to harmony.

For some, health seems to be a natural state that has come easily and is rarely lost. These people may just be lucky, or perhaps they have been blessed with certain gifts. However, can we create our own luck and destiny? How much of our health is governed by genetic factors, environmental, societal factors? What about karmic factors? It is said that there is a universal law related to action and reaction. This is referenced, in some form, in all our different religious texts. Almost all of us are familiar with the quote, "As you sow, so shall you reap." It this law of action and reaction, that is one of the cornerstones at the foundation of most religious teachings. It assists us in our determination of right from wrong. "Do unto others as you would have others do unto you," is a guiding universal principle. Many seek to honor this in their actions if for no other reason than to avoid some possible retribution occurring at a future time. "What goes around comes around," is just another variation on the theme. Yet, even if there are aspects of our own individual health status that are destined or which we may have been conscious or unconsciously responsible for creating, there remains for us a free will zone. It is here where we can exert influence on that destiny. It is a realm where we can actively work with our intention to create a new and different reality for our future. We need not be limited to our past expectations and belief systems. We can, through our choices, take actions that have both an affect and effect on our lives. Perhaps there is a portion of our life's journey that cannot be changed and charts the course for our essential life themes, events, and issues. Some have used the analogy of the major karmic experience being like train station stops in our life journey. How we lay the track between those major stations is our free will zone and it is our actions in this realm, which then go on to lay the seeds for our future experiences. Some of those past actions, thoughts, or deeds, have brought us to this moment providing us with the life circumstances, genetic makeup, and environmental surroundings for our existence. Innumerable others reside unseen, awaiting formation of our future experiences yet to come.[3]

When it comes to our health, karmic issues may be affecting us. However, one should never underestimate the effects our actions, choices, and free will have on our current life circumstances. The interplay of the karmic forces along with our current actions, thoughts, words, and deeds create our future. With the proper harnessing of one's intention and a focus on what it is that we want to create in our life, we have power to affect change and transformation. Our intention affects not only our own individual existence but ultimately it is intertwined with, and affects, that of the entire creation. We can be healed and become whole again. Where there is breath there is life, and where there is life there is hope!

Certain priorities may take precedent when one is ill. Illness can occur on different and/or simultaneous levels. One can be physically ill, emotionally ill, and/or spiritually ill. Sometimes circumstances, seemingly outside of our control, catapult our growth to a new way of thinking, feeling, and being. Sometimes the confrontation with our illness serves as the catalyst that ignites our growth. I have worked with patients going through a health crisis that found the impetus and inspiration to make conscious changes in their belief systems that altered not only their habits, lifestyle behaviors, and choices, but their entire life's course. These changes can encompass many aspects: diet, exercise, career, relationship, thought patterns, habits, and spiritual awareness, etc. An apparent or seemingly physical body health problem sometimes will not resolve unless the actions taken address underlying core emotional or spiritual health issues. Such issues may silently reside at the root and core center of our "dis-ease," insidiously undermining all that we are seeking to attain. We are such unique entities, with the integration of so many complex components. Sometimes, what seems so obvious is but an illusion.

Just as we may organize our life with a daily list of tasks to be accomplished, with a hierarchy of priorities from the most important to the least, or from the easy to the most difficult, there are priority systems that operate in both obvious and invisible ways regarding our body and our overall health. Is one in better health to be a good physical specimen but emotionally or spiritually crippled? Or, is one healthier being limited in one's capability to perform in realms of the physical, yet are emotionally and/or spiritually vital and dynamic? Ultimately, we have to determine what it is that we seek in life and determine our priorities. We have but a limited time allotted us now at this time. As it has been said, "Who knows, we might not rise from our beds to see tomorrow's dawn!"

As we continue to mature on life's journey, we come to realize that the events that have occurred are not of themselves good or bad. They simply provide us an opportunity for our continued evolution. With each choice we make, we can examine whether we are becoming more "sound," and moving into "light," and on to health and wholeness, or whether we are moving away. What foods do we eat? What are our thoughts? How do we act and behave toward others? Do we exercise? Are we kind? Are we truthful? How much and what is it we drink? Are our work and leisure activities supporting us in the attainment of our goals? Are we being conscious in our living moment to moment? Do we only take what life has to give, or do we give freely of ourselves to life? All of these things and innumerable others have all contributed to bring us to our current state—where we are right now, in this present moment. The choices that we make today affect not only our ability to move into the future but affect where we will be tomorrow.

Meditation: From Healing to Wholeness

If one were to consider the documented physical benefits that have been directly attributed to meditation practices, there would be reason enough to motivate one's pursuit of a regular routine of meditation into daily life. There are so many studies that have now linked meditation to the beneficial health effects of: decreasing blood pressure, slowing of the heart rate, reducing the deleterious effects of stress, reducing cellular damage, etc. Numerous books published have provided simple and effective forms of meditation practices for the enhancement of one's physical and emotional health. In Benson's seminal 1975 book, *The Relaxation Response*, the Harvard professor was one of the first to scientifically document those benefits related to meditation.

However, what if there were reasons to meditate even more valuable then seeking to improve one's physical and emotional health? What if there was another critical dimension to the practice of meditation? What if a meditation practice could reconnect one to their spiritual source at the heart of their being? What if the metaphysical concept of a Universal Intelligence that has created and sustains the creation does have a direct link with the spirit we are that animates our physical body? What if, analogous to Palmer's theory of removing blockages and interference to a physical body through a "chiropractic adjustment," it was possible through a "spiritual adjustment" to open the door to our spirit's connection to this force, capable of promoting our spiritual growth, evolution, and ultimate wholeness? What if we had a specific meditation practice that enabled us to have a conscious experience of that Universal Intelligence? What if the spiritual adjustment enabled one to connect, commune, and ultimately reunite to that universal power and then merge back into that creative essence from whence it emanated?

Just as a "Master" chiropractor knows how to locate and remove the interference that is adversely affecting the physical health of an individual, a true "Master" in the art of meditation could remove the interference that was adversely affecting our spiritual health. As there are gradations of competency in all fields, so too is it in this field as well. A chiropractic physician able to locate interference in the physical body and correctly treat it at the highest priority level can provide the catalyst to the physical body for healing and a return to wholeness. In the realm of the spiritual, it functions in a similar manner. A meditation Master of the highest order is able to provide us a personal inner experience through specialized focused meditation techniques enabling us to connect with the universal spiritual essence within ourselves. Once the process has begun we are able to continue to make progress, ever clarifying our experience of spirit as we merge ever deeper into our essential self, advancing us on the incredible journey back to our Source!

There are Masters of meditation capable to perform the essential spiritual "adjustment" required that can unlock our human potential and destiny.[4] It is the ability of these meditation Masters, who are themselves attuned and consciously connected to this divine universal intelligence energy, to provide one the "spiritual adjustment" so that we too are able to connect, experience, and unify with it within our own body.

One needs diligence, effort, and grace to succeed in our quest to be healed and to regain our wholeness. With our health maximized, we can best pursue the wonders and mysteries of life, seeking our ultimate destiny. In chiropractic care, the proof is in the experience of one's own physical healing process; overcoming pain, dysfunction, and disability. In meditation, the proof is in the experience of one's own process of spiritual healing.

Scientific research continues to study, evaluate, and better understand chiropractic, healing, meditation, and consciousness. We are ever learning more about this incredible body in which we reside and the essential role that chiropractic and meditation play. With every new step forward, we progress closer to the manifestation of a "golden age" of awareness, bringing our physical existence on earth ever closer to a harmonious relationship with that of the spiritual and the divine.

Sometimes it is the cry of our body that must be heard so the door to our physical healing can be opened. Sometimes it is the cry of our soul that must be heard so the door to our spirit's healing can be revealed. It is through the harmonization of our physical with the spiritual that we can again become one. It is through meditation that we can experience the ultimate zenith of existence, the union of our soul with the essence of creation.

Alan R. Post, D.C. is a chiropractic physician with a Bachelor of Science in Human Biology. Dr. Post graduated with honors from Logan College of Chiropractic in 1982 and has postgraduate certification in acupuncture. In 1993, he was a member of the North American Physician Delegation to China through the International Academy of Clinical Acupuncture. He is a past president of both Rhode Island state & North-East regional chiropractic associations. He is a member on the Advisory Board at the University of Bridgeport Chiropractic College. Dr. Post has instructed physicians for continuing education credentialing and is an integrative medicine program consultant. He has been active in health care reform, participating on numerous committees as both a member and a presenter. Dr. Post maintains two active patient care practices in Rhode Island. He has received numerous awards for his professional service.

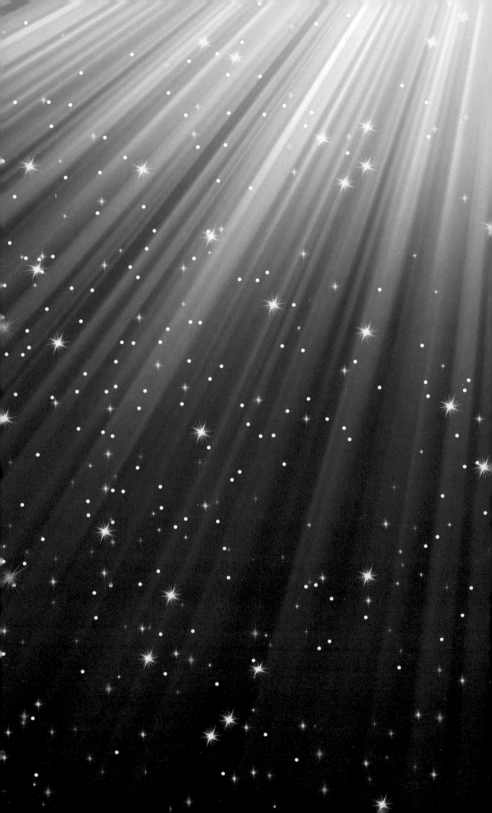

PART 5

Meditation
and
the Brain

CHAPTER 12

NEUROTHEOLOGY: THE BRAIN AND THE SCIENCE OF MEDITATION

by Louis A. Ritz, Ph.D.

**Department of Neuroscience,
University of Florida College of Medicine**

Spirituality and meditation are being increasingly embraced around the world, including the West, as our lives are becoming more and more complex. Individuals are turning within themselves, instead of the outside world, to find solutions to life's challenges. Spirituality is gaining popularity for a variety of reasons, e.g., a search for deeper meaning, dealing with unbridled emotions or an unruly mind, a fear of death, a fear of life, a loss of a loved one, or a health challenge. At a deeper level, there is a common source of our suffering. As each of us becomes more entangled in the impermanence of the outer world, our level of dissatisfaction and disappointment with everyday life inevitably rises. Instead of identifying with our true Self deep within, as the great Teachers from all wisdom traditions have implored us, our attention and intentions have remained aligned with the illusory self and the ephemeral outside world. Ironically, it is our suffering that propels many of us to inculcate spirituality into our lives.

While the impermanent world swirls around each of us, creating challenges and disharmony in our lives, there is an accessible still-point of bliss deep within. As Mark Nepo (2006), a spirituality author and cancer survivor, states: "Each person is born with an unencumbered spot, free of expectation and regret, free of ambition and embarrassment, free of fear and worry, an umbilical spot of grace where we were first touched by God." The spiritual techniques to access and experience such a still-point of bliss, "an umbilical spot of grace," include meditation and prayer. Meditation, a cornerstone of spirituality, is considered to be humanity's panacea in that it allows us to reconnect with the Divine that is within each of us (Singh, Rajinder, 2007a, 2007b, 2011).

Increasingly, the techniques of meditation are falling under the microscope of Western medical science as investigators are exploring brain mechanisms, and health benefits, associated with meditation. There is growing interest in "Neurotheology," which can be considered the role of the brain in the *experience* of God. This definition implies going beyond an intellectual study of God. To introduce Neurotheology and the science of meditation, this chapter will briefly summarize: 1) the scientific studies of meditation's influence on the body and brain, 2) the general arena of health benefits of meditation, 3) the scientific approach to employing meditation in our daily lives, and 4) the transcendent mechanisms, invoked during meditation, which might extend beyond the brain. The unique approach of this chapter, regarding the issue of the brain's role in meditation and spiritual experiences, is to discuss both brain and "trans-brain" mechanisms involved in our experiences of the Divine.

1) Scientific Studies of Meditation and the Brain
"The Physiology of Meditation"

While yoga and meditation have been investigated by scientists since the 1930s, it can be said that the modern era of scientific exploration began with the physiological studies of Robert Wallace and Herbert Benson on Transcendental Meditation (TM) (Wallace, 1971; Wallace and Benson, 1972). In their physiological evaluations, they found that during TM there were decreases in heart rate, cardiac output, blood pressure, oxygen consumption, and carbon dioxide elimination. In addition, there were increases in skin resistance. These observations led the investigators to conclude that meditation induces a "hypometabolic" state, a physiological state distinct from waking, sleeping, or dreaming.

The investigators speculated that TM, through as yet unrevealed mechanisms, influences the brain's hypothalamus and brainstem to bring about changes in metabolism and physiological functions. However meditation induces these changes in brain functions, it appears that in a hypometabolic state the parasympathetic ("rest and digest") portion of the autonomic nervous system is activated and the sympathetic ("fight or flight") portion is inactivated. It is likely that these mechanisms are invoked by all meditation techniques of a tranquil nature.

Brain-Based Experiences

In 1997, two neurologists from UCLA, Dr. Jeff Saver and Dr. John Rabin, published an academic publication "The Neural Substrates of Religious Experiences," which speculated on brain mechanisms related to hallucinogenic drugs, near-death experiences, and temporal lobe epilepsy. The article begins with the definitive statement: "Religious experience is brain-based." The authors continued, expanding on their treatise: "This should be taken as an unexceptional claim. All human experience is brain-based, including scientific reasoning, mathematical deduction, moral judgment, and artistic creation, as well as the religious states of mind." Most brain scientists and clinicians would probably agree with such a position. Perhaps others, with an expanded appreciation of the complexity of human experiences, would offer a minority report. That is, some scientists are left to conclude that human experience cannot be solely reduced to the functions of brain circuits.

As we further explore these issues below, it will be argued that religious/spiritual experiences can involve both brain and "trans-brain" mechanisms. That is, sensory/motor events of the physical domain are mediated by the physical brain. Transcendent experiences, beyond the physical domain (and the physical brain), require different, subtler mechanisms that will be described below.

Meditation and the Frontal Lobes

A survey of the cerebral cortex of humans (Nadeau et al., 2004) indicates that specific regions are dedicated to specific sensory-motor functions. For example, the primary visual cortex is in the occipital lobe, the primary somatosensory cortex is in the parietal lobe, the primary motor cortex is in the frontal lobe, and the primary auditory cortex is in the temporal lobe. Note, however, that the primary cortices make up only 15% of the cerebral cortex. The remaining 85% of the cerebral cortex are involved in what are referred to as "higher cortical functions," functions beyond primary sensory-motor responsibilities. Such higher functions include the sensory and motor aspects of language, storage and retrieval of memories, higher order processing of sensory information, and higher order planning of motor activities. The frontal lobes, considered to be the executor of the highest human activities, are associated with personality, expectations and planning, motivation, attention, and social adaptations. From the vast behavioral repertoire of the frontal lobes, their role in meditation is a logical target for investigation.

The left frontal lobe, in particular, has been targeted by investigators regarding its role in happiness and other positive emotions (Davidson, 2004; Lutz et al., 2008). Neurologists are familiar with behavioral deficits caused by cerebrovascular disease or damage to the left frontal lobes. These unfortunate individuals are limited in their experience of the joyfulness of life. Recently, investigators have targeted the left frontal lobe with transcranial magnetic stimulation in cases of severe depression (George, 2010). Activation of this region was beneficial to a significant number of patients. Recent neuroimaging studies have summarized the initial evidence indicating the involvement during meditation of fronto-limbic circuits for emotional control and of fronto-parietal connections for attentional processing (Rubia, 2009; Slagter et al., 2011).

Neurotheoplasticity: Changing the Brain from Within

Some neuroscientific research regarding the impact of meditation on the brain involves H.H. the Dalai Lama. In recent years he has had provocative and insightful meetings with prominent neuroscientists to explore the intersection of the brain and the mind. Susan Begley's 2007 book entitled *Train your Mind, Change your Brain* chronicles discussions on the cutting-edge topic of neuroplasticity.

Neuroplasticity means that the brain can be shaped, or sculpted, by experiences of the external world. Until recent times, neuroscientists assumed that the mature brain is hard-wired. That is, once neural circuits are established, there is no reorganization – regardless of injury, disease, or aging. When a neural circuit is disrupted or destroyed, it is not replaced and as a result a specific function is typically lost. Yet over the past 20 years or so, a new set of rules has emerged for central nervous system organization and reorganization. Stem cells in the adult brain are a potentially important aspect of neuroplasticity. Our understanding of the mechanisms of regeneration of central nervous system fiber tracts, after injury, is rapidly expanding. The cellular mechanisms of memory formation, through strengthening of synaptic connections, are better understood. The brain definitely displays plasticity.

It is also clear that experiences of the outer world can change the circuits of the brain. For example, improvements in motor skills are accompanied by an increase in size of the brain regions related to the motor skill. Less well appreciated is how inner, or spiritual, experiences can alter the brain. The generalized process of neuroplasticity might be expanded to include the specialized process of "neurotheoplasticity." While most studies of neuroplasticity are focused on the interaction of the outer, or objective, world with the brain, nascent investigations of neurotheoplasticity center on how our inner, or subjective, world can impact the brain. How the inner process of spiritual development manifests as changes in the physical brain is currently in the early stages of understanding. The research from Dr. Richard Davidson's lab, cited above, has been inspired by H.H. the Dalai Lama.

One hint of how our inner landscape can affect our brain is demonstrated in a study of structural changes in the brain in some meditators (Lazar et al., 2005). These investigators compared the brains of two age-matched groups, one group being meditators and the other being non-meditators. Using magnetic resonance imaging (MRI) to measure the thickness of cortical areas of the brain, there were significant differences in the thickness of areas associated with meditation. Of special interest is that brain atrophy, which takes place as a normal part of aging, was reduced in the meditators. While interpretation of this study must proceed cautiously, it is an exciting first step in understanding "how the inside changes the outside." More recently, Holzel et al., (2010)

evaluated the impact of the 8-week Mindfulness-Based Stress Reduction program on brain cortical structure. A key feature of this study, in contrast to the prior investigation, is that the subjects were imaged before and after the 8-week program. The subjects had significant increases in the hippocampus and in the cingulate gyrus, which are important for memory formation and emotional regulation. By embracing spirituality and meditation, we can change our thought patterns and our brain circuits, which in turn will change our behaviors and our lives.

"Why God Won't Go Away"

Andy Newberg, a neuroradiologist from the University of Pennsylvania, is a leader in the scientific research associated with brain imaging of spiritual experiences. His efforts have been documented in his book, co-authored by Eugene d'Aquili, *Why God Won't Go Away: Brain Science and the Biology of Belief.* Newberg and his colleagues have imaged Buddhist monks in meditation and Franciscan nuns deep in devotional prayer. Using PET scans of the contemplator's brains, blood flow through the brain was monitored during the exercise. (Blood flow increases to a brain region active during a task, and decreases to a brain region inactive during a task.) Individuals in each group, during their contemplation, signaled the experimenters when s/he reached a state of "union with the universe." Significantly, during this spiritual experience there was a decrease in blood flow to the right parietal lobe. In stroke victims, lesions of this brain region lead to "hemispatial neglect," in which the patient is unaware of the left portion of their spatial world. Apparently, during the contemplative practice, the diminished activity of the right parietal lobe (and, perhaps the left parietal lobe) is correlated with a loss of awareness of the physical world – interpreted as an experience of Divine merger. Newberg believes that strong evidence of the brain's involvement in these spiritual experiences is indicative of a connection between humans and God. Indeed, this is the reason for Newberg's belief in why God will not go away. God has provided humans with brain circuits that allows us to experience the Divine.

The Mystical Experiences of Carmelite Nuns

Beauregard et al. (2006, 2007, and 2008) investigated the neural circuits involved in the mystical union, born of contemplative practices, experienced by Carmelite nuns. These scientific studies were unique in that the nuns were attempting to have, or at least remember and relive, a mystical experience involving a union with the Creator. Imaging studies with fMRI (functional MRI) and electrophysiological analyses of EEG were correlated with qualitative evaluations of the subjective experiences of the nuns. Of note, many areas of the brain, including the frontal lobes, parietal lobes, basal ganglia, and brainstem, were activated during the session. The authors concluded that there is no single region in the brain dedicated to spiritual experiences.

Summary of the Brain's Role in Religious/Spiritual Experiences

The body's brain is the crown jewel of *physical creation*, the control center of the physical body; the brain's domain is the physical realm but not beyond. The brain, as a first approximation, receives sensory impressions from the world and generates the motor signals that will move the body's muscles. Thus, all religious/spiritual experiences of a *physical nature* including visual, auditory, and emotional experiences will be mediated by the physical brain. It appears that brain correlates of religious/spiritual experiences are, in general, distributed across several of the brain's circuits that are associated with our typical sensory, motor, attentional, and emotional activities. However, subjective experiences of a mystic, which are found beyond the physical domain, will of necessity require mechanisms beyond the physical brain. These mechanisms will be discussed at the end of the chapter.

2) The Health Benefits of Meditation

In this section, we will highlight: i) the role of meditation as a complementary medicine—that of facilitating our wellness and of complementing Western, allopathic medicine when needed; ii) the 12-Step Program as a spiritual intervention for the health program of addiction; and, iii) how meditation can reduce stress in our lives.

Meditation: The Ultimate Complementary Medicine

Over the past decade, there has been a burgeoning interest in alternative medicines in general and in meditation specifically. A 2002 survey, conducted by Dr. David Eisenberg's research team from Harvard Medical School (Tindle et al.,2005), documents that Americans are increasingly embracing complementary and alternative medicine, including meditative techniques. There are numerous reasons that people embrace meditation—to relieve stress, to stop the chattering mind, to calm the volatile emotions, to remove the superficial masks of our lives, or to facilitate the search for meaning in life and connection with a higher power. A National Health Statistics Report (Barnes et al., 2008), commissioned by the Centers for Disease Control and Prevention, indicates that 9.4% of Americans have incorporated meditation, in some form, into their lives.

Meditation—with the ability to impact the physical body, the emotions, the mind, and the soul—can be considered the ultimate complementary medicine. This is not to imply that meditation can necessarily cure the major physical diseases afflicting humans. It can, however, provide significant relief by altering one's perspective regarding the physical malady and by reducing stress that exacerbates physical problems and impedes healing. It is supremely effective, when properly applied, for deeper, more complex, problems of disorderly emotions and mental activity.

The highest impetus to incorporate meditation into our lives is the search for the Sacred within, the pinnacle of life according to the saints and mystics (Singh, Rajinder, 2007a, 2007b, 2011). Meditation, as a process for delving into our own inner silence and darkness, facilitates the emergence of divine vistas and sounds. In the process, our number one health (and spiritual!) challenge is confronted—that of our separation from the Creator. All other spiritual/health issues devolve from this separation. That is, the subsequent karmic reactions to our on-going actions, since this long-ago separation, are considered to be the root causes of the various physical and emotional health problems that each of us faces.

Meditation can be regarded as the ultimate complementary medicine due to the breath of its impact on a human being. Not only are there spiritual benefits, but also psychological and physical. These diverse, positive benefits are eloquently stated by Dr. Roger Walsh, author of *Essential Spirituality*—"The ultimate aim of spiritual practices is awakening; that is, to know our true Self and our relationship to the sacred. However, spiritual practices also offer numerous other gifts along the way...the heart begins to open, fear and anger melt, greed and jealousy dwindle, happiness and joy grow, love flowers, peace replaces agitation, concern for others blossoms, wisdom matures, and both psychological and physical health improve..."

Another reason that meditation can be considered the ultimate complementary medicine has to do with the lifestyle in which the meditative experience is embedded. Just like an athlete's lifestyle must be consistent with the individual's athletic goals, so too a meditator's lifestyle must resonate with his or her spiritual goals. Athletes do not just spend a few hours a day in training. They must also be concerned with their diet, their interactions with others, and their priorities. Similarly, meditation does not have to be an isolated activity done only for a set length of time each day. When coupled with an ethical approach to living, meditation can be expanded to a "24/7" lifestyle commitment. Many choose to couple meditation with an outer ethical life that includes the loving virtues of humility, non-violence, truthfulness, purity of heart, and selfless service. Far from limiting our lives, it has been said that these virtues can be thought of as life preservers that keep us from drowning in the stormy oceans of worldly life. As such, the meditator can choose to live a lifestyle that is physically and psychologically healthy in all aspects.

The 12-Step Program

While our intent here is not to have an in-depth discussion of addiction, the 12-Step Program represents a potent therapeutic intervention that demonstrates the link between spirituality and health. Alcoholism is a vexing problem that has plagued humankind for centuries. It is becoming more evident, in recent years, that there may well be a biological basis for alcoholism and other drug addictions. The brain circuitry of addiction involves the so-called "reward pathway" or "pleasure pathway." It appears that most addictive, chemical substrates directly or indirectly activate this pathway to generate an exaggerated subjective experience of pleasure or reward—ultimately at a huge cost to the individual.

162

The 12-Step Program is a spiritual intervention, considered to be the most effective self-help program dealing with addiction. The major spiritual aspects of the 12-Step Program include acknowledgement of the need for a higher Power (however defined by an individual), humility, atonement for shortcomings, infusion of prayer and meditation into the lifestyle, and—as a natural outcome of spiritual development—service to others struggling with the same malady. The appropriate cure is not simply a detoxification, but a transformation of an individual based on spiritual action. While addiction is a biologically-based disease, like diabetes, it can be confronted with a spiritual solution. Similar to diabetes, the disease can be managed on a daily basis with a spiritual outlook. Indeed, it might be argued that many of our physical health concerns have a spiritual answer. While psychosomatic therapies are familiar to us, addiction requires something that reaches even deeper—what we might call "theosomatic interventions" (Levin, 2002). It is suggested that the power of the soul supersedes the efficacy of the brain's network of neurons that are a biological factor in addiction. The power of the soul can best be invoked by meditation (Singh, Rajinder, 2007b).

Meditation and Stress Reduction

The work of Jon Kabat-Zinn and Saki Santorelli, over the past 30 years, has introduced meditation to many Americans including the medical establishment (e.g., Kabat-Zinn, 2005; Santorelli, 2000). They have promoted the daily use of meditation, with focus on the breath, and, as important, a lifestyle of living "in the moment." Their approach is called mindfulness.

Mindfulness, being present, living in the moment, however named, is a component of every contemplative practice of our wisdom traditions. It is, in fact, not possible to focus on the sacred within if we are focusing out of the present (i.e., in the past or future). Self-introspection of the mind's activities, during our contemplative practice, will quickly indicate to the practitioner the issues and melodramas that are taking him or her out of the present. Armed with this awareness, the practitioner can adjust his lifestyle to minimize or eliminate the distraction. While meditation is a period of time when we devote ourselves wholly and solely to focusing inward, keeping our attention on the present is also important throughout our everyday life.

The role of the mind, in the grand scheme of things, is said to keep us out of the present moment, the "now," by taking us into the past or the future. These concepts of time are constructs of the mind. It is our mental sojourns into the past or future that generate and reinforce our worries, anxieties, fear, guilt, remorse, and uncertainties—the key components of stress. Stress seems to be associated with every health challenge, either by causing the health problem or by making it worse. By causing the chronic release of "stress hormones," which have deleterious consequences to our cardiovascular system, stress can be very insidious. This is an unfortunate consequence of the "mind-body" connection.

It can, in fact, be argued that stress is self-inflicted. By considering whether stress is a "cause" or an "effect," it should become apparent that stress is a result of our psychological reaction to events of the outside world. These events, which can be called challenges or opportunities, are in fact neutral experiences. That is, it is we who determine, by our internal reactions, whether an event is stressful. It has been suggested that we "don't react" to life's incidents, at least with a knee-jerk psychological reflex. "Don't react" is a simple but powerful adage to help us control our stress, thus benefiting our health. Meditation can help us decouple the automatic stimulus-response mechanism by making us more aware of our reactions to the challenges of life.

3) The Scientific Approach to Meditation

Meditation is, more and more, falling under the microscope of scientific investigation. Indeed, the phrase "Science of Meditation" can be found on the covers of two popular magazines, *Time* (August 4, 2003) and *Scientific American Mind* (February/March 2006). What does the "Science of Meditation" imply? Spiritual questions, like medical or other scientific questions, can be investigated with rigorous, systematic techniques using the time-honored scientific method. Whether an individual is using the scientific method to investigate the objective outer world or the subjective inner realms, the technique is equally valid and valuable.

Use of the scientific method as a guideline for spiritual exploration has been developed and promoted by the great spiritual scientists of modern times. The basic spiritual questions, that have crossed many minds, as our lives and fates are pondered, include: "Who are we? Why are we here? Where are we going when we leave here? And, what is our relationship to the Creator?" The spiritual explorers have long considered these questions to be answerable through personal spiritual inquiry; however, unlike objective research questions, they require us to conduct experiments for ourselves, within ourselves.

The following steps are required for a scientific approach to meditation, within the context of the experimental paradigm. Such a paradigm, when exploring our spiritual nature, can be considered in the following manner.

1) Entering a new field of scientific study requires guidance from an experienced researcher. Like graduate school or medical school, in which the students are required to have a research mentor, spirituality also offers such a relationship. A budding research endeavor requires an experienced guide. For our spiritual research the guidance of an appropriate mentor, who has mastered the spiritual journey, is beneficial. People have

mentors throughout their lifetimes, for help with learning to speak, to navigate adolescence, to drive a car, or to prepare for a profession. Spirituality, the greatest and most challenging of human endeavors, likewise offers the help of a mentor.

2) Scientific research begins with questions. Subsequently, the questions crystallize into a testable hypothesis. (Questions with no answers, that are not testable, fall out of the realm of scientific exploration.) Our spiritual research is not approached willy-nilly, but is propelled by our initial questions. For example, one may hypothesize that a person can have an experience of divine light or inner vistas. It is the spiritual advisor who helps us define our spiritual research project.

3) The techniques for data collection, which will allow us to accept or to reject our hypothesis, are taught to us by the mentor. The mentor gives guidance in at least five domains:

    i. He teaches his mentees the proper techniques to answer their questions and achieve their goals;

    ii. He provides the best shortcuts to achieve progress with our scientific technique;

    iii. He provides us with ancillary suggestions, such as focusing on spirituality through reading books, listening to audio or watching video on spiritual topics, attending spiritual gatherings or satsangs, or completing daily the diary form, that will enhance the efficacy of our scientific approach;

    iv. He alerts the aspirant to potential pitfalls along the journey; and,

    v. He helps us monitor our progress.

4) In order to conduct an experiment in a proper scientific fashion, a laboratory is required. In the case of the spiritual investigation, the human body is our laboratory (Singh, Rajinder, 2005). However, laboratories in modern research facilities are typically locked. The human laboratory, similarly, has a blocked passageway that can only be unblocked by the spiritual adept. This opening is done at the time of initiation into meditation on

light and sound within.

5) To collect our data, in order to accept or reject our spiritual hypothesis, we must use the delicate instruments of the spiritual laboratory. In a sophisticated medical research facility, a fledgling student does not walk into a laboratory and immediately use the equipment. Similarly, a neophyte spiritual aspirant can receive guidance from the spiritual mentor, who teaches the aspirant to use properly the laboratory's instruments — the inner eye and inner ear. In addition, the mentor delineates an outer ethical lifestyle that will reinforce and promote the inner exploration.

No scientific progress is made without a lot of hard work, without patience, without perseverance, which help to perfect the experiment. Similarly, these attributes are important for us to progress spiritually. When we conduct a scientific experiment, we need to be fully focused on the task at hand, to perform the experiment with precision. In a similar vein, our mentor encourages us to approach the spiritual experiment with accuracy, steadfastness, and absorption.

6) Following an experiment in a medical institute, observations and data are collected on a computer or in a journal. Similarly, after one's spiritual experiment, the results are recorded. The results of our efforts are recorded in an introspection diary form, to note progress. The spiritual diary form was devised by Sant Kirpal Singh Ji Maharaj, and recommended by Sant Rajinder Singh Ji Maharaj, to aid in one's scientific exploration of the spiritual realms. One can track the trends of our thoughts, words, and deeds to help us be more aware of the roadblocks to a successful spiritual experiment.

7) In the best of medical research situations, the experiments are repeated daily until the techniques are perfected; the process of science is iterative. In the spiritual experiment there also must be repetition — one meditates daily.

8) Typically, in a medical research lab, the mentor periodically reviews the progress of the students. Refinement of one's spiritual techniques with the help of the spiritual mentor is a necessary step in one's spiritual development. Such feedback may come during a personal interaction with the mentor or in written form; in any case, the advice can speed one's progress.

9) The final step of the scientific process is to communicate one's results. In the medical world, this may be done with a presentation at a scientific conference or through publication in a respected scientific journal. In the spiritual domain, the outcome of our experiments will be an individual with an empowered and emboldened soul—one who exhibits an approach to life displaying blissfulness, connectedness, fearlessness, immortality, wisdom, and unconditional love (Singh, Rajinder, 2007b).

A scientific model of meditation will provide the aspirant with a rigorous, reproducible approach to the practice of meditation. The steps involved in meditation will allow the fledging spiritual scientist to enjoy physical and psychological benefits and enrichments that extend beyond our physical frame.

4) Experiences beyond the Physical Body/ Brain "Encased in our Spacesuits"

The following is a simple, and incomplete, analogy meant to highlight and emphasize the various layers of a human being. Our story starts with an individual who leaves home, where he existed unencumbered and untethered, to travel to a far-off planet. The conditions on this planet are such that the person needs a spacesuit in order to exist, interact with, and survive in the new environment. After some time, our traveler leaves the first planet for another destination, again requiring an additional spacesuit for the new locale, with the new suit overlying and intermingling with the original suit. Again, at a later time, the individual leaves for a third planet, which demands the use of a third spacesuit. The explorer is now covered by three spacesuits, co-existing, all required to exist in this final domain. After some time, the outer spacesuit wears out and the astronaut is required to return to the second locale (with but two spacesuits on). And so the story goes.

A human being is more, much more, than the physical frame. According to the spiritual teachers, saints, and sages, we all are like our traveler. Our soul left its true home sometime in the distant past, the region of pure spirit and consciousness, for the first destination. In this supracausal realm, a thin covering was required. In the next region, the causal realm, an appropriate spacesuit is required – the causal body. Subsequently, the soul heads for the next destination, the astral realm, and another appropriate spacesuit is mandated—the astral body—so it can function in this new environment. At this point, the soul is surrounded by three spacesuits, coverings, or bodies (supracausal, causal, and astral). For the final destination, the physical realm far from the home base, yet another spacesuit is necessary—the physical body. As before, at this point the traveler is encased with four functional and interactive spacesuits, constituting our supracausal veil, our causal body, our astral body, and our physical body. When the outer suit is no longer functional and must be discarded (i.e., at the time of death), the traveler returns to the astral realm surrounded by the supracausal veil and the causal and the astral body, but no longer the physical senses. The inner journey continues from there.

With the techniques espoused by the Masters of Sant Mat, during meditation the attention (surat) is shifted from one body to the next, i.e., from the physical body to the astral body. Normally, as we are embodied in the physical frame, our attention is scattered throughout the body and the physical world, as dictated by the mind and its cohort the senses. In the process of meditation, the senses are inactivated by shutting out the outside world. With the help of a competent teacher, by focusing the attention at the third eye, as described above, one can begin to withdraw from the physical realm and experience lights and sounds of the realms beyond.

An apt analogy given by Sant Rajinder Singh Ji is to consider our brain to be like a cable box for our TV. As such, our brain is receptive to many different "channels." We can set it to watch the channel of the physical world, the channel of the body, the channel of the emotions, or the channel of the mind. Most of us spend our entire lives experiencing one of these four channels, with the mind probably occupying most of our attention. A few of us may, with good fortune, explore another channel available to each of us on our cable box—the "channel of God" (Singh, Rajinder, 2005). We can begin to tune into this channel of God by focusing our attention at the third eye (or sixth chakra) between and behind the eyebrows. This channel is so subtle and so faint, at least at first, that it requires special tuning of our attention— through an ethical lifestyle and meditation. With loving attention focused at the third eye, we can begin to experience inner realms.

"Trans-Brain" Mechanisms of Religious/Spiritual Experiences

To some, the summary in previous sections of the chapter would suffice to explain the role of the central nervous system in mystical experiences, as "religious experience is brain-based" (Saver and Rabin, 1997). But to others, there are experiences that cannot be explained fully by brain circuitries and mechanisms. One such experience is a near-death experience (NDE), in which an individual following a close brush with death is transported to another realm (Moody, Raymond, 1976; Singh, Rajinder, 2007a). In this domain beyond the physical realm, bright lights, sounds, and vistas beyond our physical realm are experienced. For whatever reason, these individuals who had an NDE return to the physical realm, to complete their responsibilities in the physical realm and to tell their stories about their inner experiences. While such occurrences are seemingly out of the ordinary realm, for saints and mystics these are commonplace.

The highest goal of a human being is to be fully integrated — body, emotions, mind, and soul. Much of what we experience is based in the physical world and as such requires the use of the brain and senses. Yet, those who tap inside through meditation have the ability to transcend the physical realm and experience realms within. Those who in meditation have combined focused attention with intense yearning, trans-brain mechanisms (or what the brain is capable of doing) transport them to inner regions of light and love to begin the journey to purely spiritual realms. Propelled by a "love (that) begins in the flesh and ends in the spirit" (Singh, Darshan, 1978) and by the unyielding efforts of the spiritual Adept, our soul's attention is gracefully disentangled with the illusory physical world and, through mechanisms extending well beyond the neural circuitry of the brain, obtains the innermost reaches of God's creation.

Louis A. Ritz, Ph.D. is on the faculty of the Department of Neuroscience within the University of Florida College of Medicine. His research interests investigated new techniques aimed at alleviating the devastating consequences of injury to the spinal cord. In recent years, Dr. Ritz has focused on medical and graduate education. He is the course director for Medical Neuroscience, taken by first year medical students. He was selected, based on an Educational Portfolio, as a member of the College of Medicine's "Society of Teaching Scholars" in 2006. At the University of Florida, he also is Director of a campus-wide Center for Spirituality and Health, which offers workshops, academic programs, and interdisciplinary research ventures exploring the impact of spirituality on health.

CHAPTER 13

REDUCING STRESS-RELATED AILMENTS IN LEARNERS FOR PEAK PERFORMANCE

by Ricki Linksman, M.Ed.

As medical research points to the connection between stress and illnesses affecting the body and mind, they also offer solutions to reduce stress. While it may not be possible to eliminate all life's difficulties, there are some stressors that we can reduce and even prevent. One cause of stress and stress-related ailments that affects people comes from the task of learning, whether in school or at work. Students of all ages are under continual pressure. There is tension in post-graduate studies, vocational studies, or training for a job or career. Those experiences are not limited to young adults starting out in the world, but with the ever-changing economy often resulting in change or loss of jobs, adults of all ages, even in their later years, face learning a new career. Athletes, artists, musicians, and entertainers also experience stress in mastering or competing in their field. No matter what one's age or subject of study, is it possible to prevent stress and its accompanying illnesses of the body and mind? First, we will examine causes of stress in learners. Second, we will look at methods to reduce and prevent stress and stress-related ailments in learners to help them attain peak performance.

Causes of Stress in Learners of All Ages

Whether one must master academic or vocational studies, learn a new job or career, take tests, or compete in sports or other fields, stress takes its toll. Learning in itself is not stressful as the brain is wired to do so from birth. Observe infants and toddlers, whose brains are learning a tremendous amount of information, knowledge, and skills; they are happy, joyful, and playful. For the infant and toddler, learning is a natural part of their development and they soak in a tremendous amount of knowledge. For example, they learn to speak an entire language, walk, and develop all the behaviors and skills they learn from their environment and culture.

Their innate curiosity and desire to explore and learn appear more like fun and play. Then, if learning is natural, enjoyable, and fun for young children, how does stress from learning arise? Stress arises from a number of conditions and situations in which learning takes place: competition; meeting and maintaining high standards as measured on tests or performance evaluations; keeping pace with the fast rate at which information is taught; not being given the proper tools, information, or help to succeed at a subject or task; work overload; and rapid change in information, methodology, and technology. Competition for placement in superior schools and colleges can result in anxiety, panic, and fear. Meeting academic standards to advance to the next grade level or face being retained in the same grade level for another year causes stress. Honor and gifted students who must maintain their high grade point average or keep up their reputation for high achievement undergo tremendous pressure. Students who cannot keep up often are diagnosed and labeled as having a learning disability, ADD, ADHD, dyslexia, or other learning problem and are often placed in special programs, adding to their stress by giving them the feeling there is something wrong with them. This can cause learners to develop low self-esteem and lack of motivation when they are not taught strategies to help them learn or improve.

Student athletes often must practice two or three hours daily after school while trying to keep up their homework and grades lest they be cut from their team. Focus on sports achievement for schools and colleges to keep up their standings are passed along to students who often must practice daily, while trying to find time to complete their homework assignments or reports, engage in test preparation, and achieve good grades. Such pressure can result in stress-related ailments.

With new technology and information bursting on the scene daily, even those who have jobs must keep up with learning new information, or using new technological devices or software. One not only has to do one's job, but one has to relearn how to do it with new technology.

Those competing for jobs in the workplace have the stress of learning new skills, revising their resumes, being able to speak knowledgably about this new information, and waiting to hear the results, often repeatedly facing rejection. In a shrinking economy with millions out of work, stress has reached epidemic proportions.

These various stressors can manifest as physical or mental symptoms. For some, they manifest as a Monday morning stomachache when returning to school or work after a weekend of fun. Anxiety can result from having to perform at a competent level, even if one does not fully understand the subject one is studying at school, or one no longer grasps what one is supposed to do at work due to new technology or information. Take the example of medical students who studied a body of information over many years, only to face new advances in diagnosis, treatment, and medication they must suddenly learn and master when they reach their last year of medical school and must pass their final examinations. They cannot rest on the knowledge they previously mastered, but must supplement that by keeping up with the new information, adding pressure to their test preparations.

Stress affects students in college, post-graduate work, or in medical or dental schools. A study at the University of California at Berkeley revealed that 67% of graduate students had "felt hopeless at least once in the last year," while 54% felt "so depressed they had a hard time functioning." The study, sponsored by the American College Health Association, raises questions about the mental health of those dealing with the rigors of graduate school.[1]

Along with digestive disorders caused by stress, learners experience tension and migraine headaches, heart palpitations, a rise in blood pressure, muscle tension, or lowered immune systems making people susceptible to a host of illnesses. A study from Johns Hopkins University School of Medicine reports that school stress raises cholesterol levels. "The findings are consistent with the hypothesis that stress such as accompanies the first few weeks of medical school or important final examinations is accompanied by a significant mean rise in cholesterol level."[2]

Besides physical manifestations of stress, there are emotional and psychological symptoms. Some manifest their stress as depression, anxiety, phobias, fear, or panic attacks. According to a recent UCLA survey of college freshman published in an article by the National Health Ministries, college students are "feeling more overwhelmed and stressed than fifteen years ago, More than 30% of all college freshman report feeling overwhelmed—a great deal of the time."[3]

Another result of stress is depression, which affects over 19 million adults in the United States annually. Anxiety disorders affect millions of adults each year. At colleges nationwide, large percentages of college students are feeling so overwhelmed, sad, hopeless, and depressed that they are unable to function. In a recent national college health survey, 10% of college students had been diagnosed with depression. Among college students, anxiety levels have been rising since the 1950s. "In 2000, 7% of college students reported experiencing anxiety disorders within the previous year. Eating disorders affect 5-10 million women and 1 million men, with the highest rates occurring in college-aged women." According to the Centers for Disease Control and Prevention (CDC), 7.8% of men and 12.3% of women ages 18-24 report frequent mental distress—a key indicator for depression and other mental disorders.[4] As one of the solutions, the Indiana University Health Center suggests, "Spend time each day with at least one relaxation technique—imagery, daydreaming, prayer, yoga or meditation."[5]

These symptoms of emotional and psychological stress afflict students of all ages, backgrounds, ethnic groups, socio-economic groups, and cultures. Stress affects students throughout the world. According to a survey titled, "Depression among Adolescents in Taipei Area," "84.2% of the surveyed adolescents have experienced depression, 15.3% reported that they feel depressed almost every day, and 33.6% said that depression occurs to them once a week.[6] In terms of stress sources, 56.7% of them considered that their depression comes from school stress, 50.9% thought that their depression is caused by interpersonal relations, and 45.6% attributed their depression to academic tests. From the above statistics, it can be inferred that school is a source of stress for adolescents.[7]

Is there any hope to reduce and prevent stress in learners of all ages and lessen their risk of contracting stress-related illnesses that affect their physical and mental health?

Preventing Stress in Learners

Throughout my forty-year professional career as an educator and founder-director of an accelerated learning and reading institute, I have witnessed the pressure people undergo when learning any subject or field. My focus as an educator has been to improve and accelerate learner performance for people of all ages to learn any subject quickly and raise self-esteem and motivation, while reducing and preventing stress so they can enjoy learning and be successful. Through years of study and keeping up with the latest brain research, my focus has been to apply those findings to the field of education and learning. Using brain-based techniques I have developed and tested accelerated learning methods that have proven to consistently take learners who were either failing, struggling, lacking in motivation, or anxious about learning to achieve phenomenal gains in performance and confidence through reducing and preventing stress. These techniques have reduced tension and accelerated learning in people of all ages. It is usual to see results in which learners of all ages rise on an average several grade levels above their age or current performance level within on average two to eight months. Besides going from failure to success, they also develop a newfound belief in their abilities, a positive attitude, motivation, high self-esteem, and a reduction in fear and stress that previously pervaded their lives. The method combines using the hidden power of their brain to accelerate their progress, while reducing and preventing stress through meditation, relaxation techniques, and visualization.

The two-part system I use has helped learners dramatically improve achievement: a) applying the groundbreaking research on brain plasticity and how the brain works to accelerate learning, and b) using meditation techniques to reduce and prevent the stress that holds learners back from optimum performance. This powerful combination of using brain-based methods to maximize learning plus the power of meditation to help attain peak performance allows learners to tap into an inner power that can produce dramatic results.

Step 1: First, through diagnosing how one learns the best, one can find the fastest and easiest modality for taking in information, comprehending, and remembering material. Once we know how our own brain learns, comprehends, and remembers in its unique way, we can adapt the method by which we are being taught to match our fastest and most effective style of learning.

For example, people learn, remember, and comprehend in different ways. Some prefer to learn through their visual learning style, while others prefer their auditory modality. Some prefer learning through their tactile modality, while others prefer the kinesthetic learning style. While most people can learn through any modality, some have a preference of taking in information in one way over the other. When instruction is given in their preferred method, learning is easier, quicker, and more automatic. When instruction is given in our non-preferred way, learning may be more difficult, slower, and stressful. Imagine the difference between writing with your dominant hand as opposed to your non-dominant hand. What if we had to take a timed test with our non-dominant hand and our grades, test scores, or job placement depended upon our performance? How stressful would that be? One can do both, but think of how much more easily, quicker, automatically, and effectively one can write with the dominant hand, especially in a high-stakes situation.

Furthermore, some people prefer using the part of the brain that favors sequential learning and do better when instructed in a step-by-step way, while others prefer using the part of the brain that thinks more globally, and do better when presented the big picture or main idea first. Similarly, if one prefers taking in information when given in words, either orally or in writing, then that approach would help one learn more quickly and easily. Alternatively, if one prefers taking in information when given in pictures, graphics, or real-life presentations, then that approach would help one learn better and more effectively. Some people learn through a combination of approaches.

The key is that everyone learns differently. When instruction is given using a method that matches our learning preference, stress is reduced and we can learn anything quickly, better, and more easily. Imagine how stressful it would be to have to take a test in a time limit, with readable handwriting with one's non-dominant hand, as opposed to the ease of writing with your dominant hand. By finding one's fastest way of learning, we can assimilate a tremendous amount of material more quickly, comprehend it better, and remember it for application or even taking tests.[8]

Step 2: Meditation, relaxation, and visualization reduces and prevents the stress that blocks us from peak performance. Brain research has mapped out different parts of the brain that perform different functions. The frontal lobe with the cerebral cortex is used for higher-level learning, planning, and execution of tasks. Other parts of the brain deal with emotions, fear, and fight or flight reactions. Consider the difference in performance when people take tests or perform at tasks when they are focused in the part of the brain used for cognitive processing and when they are focused in the part of the brain in which they experience fear. We can better able to access cognitive information when processing in our cerebral cortex and less able to access cognitive information when in the part of the brain in which fear, panic, and the fight or flight mode are mediated. We may have experienced for ourselves, or know of top students who "cannot take a test." They may be smart, capable, and have all the knowledge within their head, but flunk the test. This phenomenon is often related to learners being so fearful of taking the test that their attention moves from their cerebral cortex where their information is stored to the part of the brain where they experience fear, panic, and anxiety during the test. Their cognitive thinking part of the brain seems to "shut down." Meditation can be an invaluable tool to help people relax during a test or performance evaluation at work so they can access the place where their information is stored. I have seen learners of all ages who have studied everything required to prepare for a test who also relaxed by meditating for a few minutes daily beginning several weeks before an exam or performance evaluation overcome their test fear.

Of course, meditation without study may not produce a raise in academic results alone; it requires a combination of both mastering information through instruction given in one's best way of learning and then meditating to be relaxed while both learning and accessing that knowledge while taking exams or performance evaluations. Meditation is a supplement to help learners achieve the results they deserve commensurate with their effort in learning and studying. These methods have consistently helped learners with a history of failure or low performance, stress, and anxiety to reach incredible heights academically, in their careers, in sports, and in many other fields. This technique has helped produce valedictorians, honor students at the top of their classes, winning athletes, and top achievers in the work place, using the combination of brain-based accelerated learning techniques and meditation to reduce and prevent stress.

In an address to the Ministry of Education in Bogota, Colombia, Sant Rajinder Singh Ji Maharaj, to whom they awarded the Medal of Cultural Merit for his work in Education and Peace, said, "There are benefits to meditation that help in our life. By meditating daily, our concentration improves. Meditation is another name for concentration. During meditation, we close our eyes and look within. What we are doing is concentrating our attention to see what lies in front of us. If we still the mind by concentration, we can use that technique in day-to-day life. Then we understand more of what we read. We complete work faster because we have developed the techniques of focusing our attention. Students do better in their studies because of improved concentration. Besides improving our intellectual abilities through meditation, we feel better physically. In meditation, we are physically relaxed. We do not become overly agitated, and our response to problems is tension-free."[9]

Along with meditation, visualization can improve performance. A study done by Alvaro Pascual-Leone, a professor of Neurology at Harvard Medical School, Director of the Berenson-Allen Center for Noninvasive Brain Stimulation, and Program Director of the Harvard-Thorndike Clinical Research Center of the Beth Israel Deaconess Medical Center in Boston, supports the power of visualization to accelerate learning. His research involves understanding the mechanisms that control brain plasticity across the lifespan so they can be modified for a learner to achieve an optimal behavioral outcome. He combines various brain imaging and brain stimulation methods to show a relationship between regional brain activation and behavior. This study involved students learning to play piano and revealed that physical changes in the brain could be brought about by thought alone. In one experiment, Alvaro Pascual-Leone taught two groups of people some basics of playing the piano. One group practiced using real pianos, while the other group practiced only in their minds. After six hours of piano practice over three days, the two groups had similar changes in their brain maps and similar improvements in actual performance. Thus, the same degree of neuron connections in the area related to playing piano was shown to have developed or grown in both groups— the group who actually played and the group that only visualized playing the piano. This demonstrates that just by imagining doing an action stimulates the same motor and sensory parts of the brain involved in doing it. Thus, we can develop our brain by just thinking and imagining ourselves doing a task. This is one graphic example of how thinking about or visualizing doing a task can result in the same brain neuron growth and connections as actually doing it.[10]

What is exciting about this study was that it confirmed scientifically through brain imaging a technique for improving comprehension, learning, and memory that proved successful in thousands of students of all ages that I have been using for decades before even such improved brain imaging was more available. If they visualized whatever they were reading as if they were actually enacting it in their mind or experienced the action in their brain, a process that I named as "virtual reality reading," they could comprehend, learn, and remember it better. By using these strategies, failing and struggling learners have consistently risen quickly to become successful, often reaching the top of the class or in their departments at work. They not only comprehended what they read, but retained it to score high on academic tests or in performance evaluations at work.

Along with this, to access that data that they read, they needed to stay out of the part of the brain in which they experience fear and go into their thinking part of their brain. This was done by 1) developing their skills along with the confidence that they knew what to do; and 2) allowing them to do meditation, relaxation, and visualization exercises.

In another study, reported in the National Academy of Sciences of the United States of America, two random groups of 45 undergraduates from the University of Oregon were divided to practice two different techniques for eleven hours of training, thirty minutes per session, over a one-month period. One group practiced a meditative technique, while the other did relaxation exercises. The brains of both groups were scanned before and after the training to analyze the white matter of the brain. The brain scans showed that there were no significant changes in the relaxation group. However, a number of areas showed significantly greater changes in the brains of the group that practiced the meditative technique.[11]

Such studies on brain plasticity and how we can strengthen brain connections through meditation open up the possibility of helping people increase learning as well as reduce symptoms of various physical and mental disorders that cause barriers for learners.

Another graphic example of the power of combining superior training, practice, and meditation comes from the world of sports. In the 1990s the championship NBA basketball team, the Chicago Bulls, was coached by Phil Jackson, nicknamed "the Zen Master." Most notable in their achievements was the amazing, almost impossible, basketball shots and performance of Michael Jordan. How did Michael Jordan do what he did and what helped Coach Phil Jackson lead the Chicago Bulls to six championships? How did Phil Jackson repeat the success with the Los Angeles Lakers, which he coached and led to five more championships? George Mumford, a sport psychologist, who worked with the Chicago Bulls, including Michael Jordan, for five years during their championship run and who later worked with the Los Angeles Lakers, described how their basketball training was supplemented with meditation. The Bulls would sit in meditation, visualize their basketball moves in their mind, and relax.[12] The result—a two three-peat champions—six championships during the time Phil Jackson and the Bulls were together. NBA finals MVP Kobe Bryant reported in a television interview held on June 17, 2009, that coach Phil Jackson had the Lakers meditate prior to games.[13] Another Lakers player, Andrew Bynum, also meditated before a game, "with a session after his pre-game lunch and shortly before the opening tip so he can visualize what's in store for later that night."[14] As Phil Jackson said in an interview about having his basketball teams meditate, "...we sit in this attitude of being able to focus and hold our attention...it is very important that they have that kind of sense of reading each other, and their level of alertness and awareness and being able to read what is going on on the court causes each of them to react in a certain way. And that's the beauty of basketball; that's the beauty of coaching."[15]

What these examples of academic success and sports achievement share in common is the formula of coupling successful training using the power of the brain combined with meditation and concentration exercises. They result in performing better, feeling more confident, increasing motivation, doing better on tests and competitions, and enjoying learning more.

Another benefit to reducing and preventing stress in learners is the overall benefit to society. Stress can often lead to anti-social behaviors, discipline problems, and increase in crime that not only affects the well-being of the individual engaging in such actions but the overall well-being of society.

In the case of academic learners, discipline problems are often a cry for help. They often stem from academic failure and frustration. Everyone wants to be successful and look good to his or her peers. When faced with the embarrassment at school of failure or of not knowing an answer, or at work by not knowing how to do a task or job, learners often use avoidance tactics to cover up their lack of knowledge. These include acting out, being a clown, avoiding work, giving up, dropping out, or getting involved with gangs or groups at work or school who engage in anti-social behaviors. I have seen many learners of all ages whose frustration at failure had led to inappropriate behaviors and discipline problems, including joining gangs. Yet, when they were given techniques to help them be successful, their bad behaviors ended and they became motivated, dedicated learners with socially accepted behaviors. This cry for help can be addressed by the two-step process: 1) Diagnose each learner's best and fastest way of learning and instruct them in their subjects or job-related skills in their own unique learning style, and 2) teach them meditation, relaxation, and visualization techniques to improve their concentration and reduce and prevent stress.

These practical applications of brain research can be used by learners of all backgrounds. The phenomenal results applied to learners in any academic setting or in the work place. These methods derive from an understanding of how the brain works and utilizing best practices to achieve successful results.

While individual cases of learners suffering from stress from learning at school or on the job are painful to watch, the sheer numbers of people experiencing these stress-related disorders worldwide are alarming. The question to ask is, does one sit back and watch these numbers of learners affected by depression, anxiety, and other physical and mental ailments continue to rise? Anyone in a position to help learners of any age may consider employing this two-step method of helping them. First, find out how they learn and adjust instruction to their unique learning style and brain style. Comprehension and memory will vastly improve, helping them deal with their various academic subjects. These techniques can also be used to help them with their sports or extracurricular activities as well. Second, show learners how meditation can reduce and prevent their stress levels from rising. By keeping them out of the fight and flight mode, it can decrease the stress-related hormones circulating through their bodies. Through teaching calming techniques, they will perform better, access their thinking part of their brain during tests or performance evaluations, and keep them free of the mental and physical disorders that arise under stress. Their concentration, performance, and physical, mental, and emotional health will improve. With the concentration they develop through meditation, their capacity to handle greater workloads can increase. They can tackle their work with calmness and balance. Work is hard enough, but bogged down by anxiety and stress, it becomes even more difficult. If we can reduce the stress in students, even with large workloads they are better able to handle it. Imagine a runner trying to run a race with the added burden of a huge weight on his or her back. Lift the weight, and he or she can run faster with less burden. If we can lift the weight of stress off learners' shoulder through helping them experience success by teaching in their best way of learning along with meditation to calm them down, they can run faster and achieve great success in their school life and in their careers.

Ricki Linksman, M.Ed. is author of numerous books on accelerated learning, reading, and improving comprehension, memory, grades, test-scores, and training for education, jobs, or careers using brain-based research, including *How to Learn Anything Quickly* (Barnes and Noble). As founder-director of an accelerated learning institute, she trains educators to accelerate learning for learners of all ages, teaches coaches to help athletes improve learning their sports, and sharing with employers techniques to help employees and professionals accelerate learning in their jobs or careers. Her award-winning programs have helped learners of all ages raise achievement years above their age within months, improve test scores and performance, and raise self-esteem and motivation. She has presented these accelerated learning methods worldwide to universities, businesses, educational institutions, and financial corporations, to professionals in the medical and legal fields, and to football, basketball, golf, and baseball coaches and sports teams.

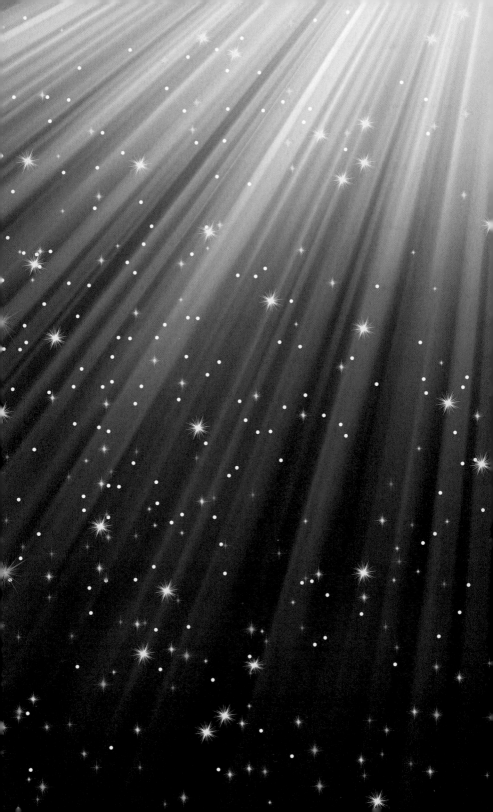

PART 6

Meditation

for

Pain

Management

CHAPTER 14

REDUCING THE PAIN OF DISABILITY THROUGH MEDITATION

By Harald Hoermann, M.S.

At a certain stage of my life, I was able to experience an intense change, a change in my way of living and my attitude towards life. I have always been a happy person, especially since I have met with my spiritual Masters, Sant Darshan Singh Ji Maharaj and Sant Rajinder Singh Ji Maharaj, and God was present in my life. I meditated regularly, and felt happy with my life. I lived in Austria and was a sports person, spending hours daily running and biking in the Austrian mountains, guiding people there and giving sports classes in the evening.

Strangely, once in a while, I had the thought, "How life would change if I would live without moving my legs." I quickly put these thoughts away finding such a thought unpleasant and unnecessary. When I thought about the consequences though, I doubted that I wanted to continue living in a situation like that, without being able to do all the sports I do, without the fun and satisfaction that derived from there and without being able to move around as freely as I did. One day seeing a person in a wheelchair I talked with a friend about it and I said that this would be the worst life situation for me. This was about one month before my life would find a dramatic change.

On my birthday, a wonderful sunny day in August, I rode my mountain bike down hills towards close-by Innsbruck University. All of a sudden, I felt my bike and myself in the air, twisting over and I found myself hitting a concrete wall with my neck and my back. Everything else is told shortly. I cannot remember the first day in the hospital before my operation, but when I woke up from the operation on my spine, I found my mother and a dear friend beside me. I could not talk but wrote down that everything was all right and that they should not worry. The doctor came and told me about my condition and that I could not walk again and that I was severely injured at my spine. This could have been the moment to make me feel really bad and sad, but…strangely…I immediately felt…my body is in pain, but for my soul, all that is happening, is a wonderful blessing. I could hardly move my head and my arms, but I felt happy inside. I felt my body is going through a hard time, but my soul is in bliss.

At the time, I already had been initiated into the method of meditation on inner light and sound in 1986 by Sant Darshan Singh Ji. Meeting Sant Darshan Singh Ji, my spiritual mentor, influenced my life tremendously in all spheres. I already had started to experience that happiness is not depending on the confines of this physical body; it comes from the spiritual realms within from where Sant Darshan Singh Ji and Sant Rajinder Singh Ji shower their unbounded love and support, lovingly and graciously, which filled me with a happiness and joy that made me want to dance in bliss.

Although I felt supported from within, I had one intense wish after the accident—I wanted to speak with Sant Rajinder Singh Ji. In the middle of the night, due to the different time zone in the United States my hospital bed was moved from the room into the corridor so as not to disturb the other patients and a phone was given to me to call Sant Rajinder Singh Ji. I was able to reach him a few hours later. One cannot imagine the waves of joy and gratitude hearing his voice on the phone. We talked for some minutes, filling me with moments of pure bliss and happiness. From then on, I felt only blessed, totally guided and extremely happy. There was no speck of sadness within me, and I shared my inner bliss and happiness with everyone around me. I have never felt so harmonious, so totally guided and one with my Masters and with God in my whole life before. I was simply happy! The pain in my body was insignificant; the joy and the feeling of being one and totally guided was overwhelming.

With deep gratitude, I thank Sant Darshan Singh Ji and Sant Rajinder Singh Ji for the grace they showered on me and still do.

As a result, I have experienced an intense amount of coping ability from being connected spiritually. As in the teachings of Sant Mat, the goal and essence of life is to grow spiritually and due to karmic processes, physical hardships can occur; these teachings helped me tremendously cope with the situation of this accident and handicap. The strong conviction that all that has happened is difficult for the body but beneficial to my soul gave me mental support and harmony in these physically difficult times. When the Masters of Sant Mat tell us that everything that happens in life is for our very best, it opens up a world of coping possibilities. In fact, I have always seen this situation of facing a physical challenge one that helped me to grow as a human being. An incident which I before had classified to be the worst thing that could happen in my life had lost its thorns and pain, and I was in a state of oneness, deep happiness, and bliss.

I may add that these intense coping processes, the feeling of joy and harmony right after my accident and in my life in a wheelchair for more than twenty years now do not only come from intellectual reasoning. Talking to friends before my accident at the sight of a person in a wheelchair, I had stated that this life situation would be the worst for me to handle. Then, a month later, facing exactly this situation, having believed it would be the worst, nevertheless finding myself in total harmony and happiness, looks like a miracle to me. I give gratitude to Sant Darshan Singh Ji, Sant Rajinder Singh Ji, and the power of God within for changing the worst situation into a source of development, connected always with much happiness and joy. To me, this is an experience of divine grace and love. These experiences of grace never stopped, but continued perpetually in my journey through life with the guidance of the Masters.

After this intense period of harmony, the work with my body and its new limitations, as well as the mental work, started with the process of rehabilitation. I experienced new challenges in how to handle my bodily functions, handle the wheelchair, and daily life.

One specific and important aspect of the spiritual path that helped me tremendously to cope with these physical and mental challenges was meditation on the inner light and sound. During rehabilitation and the following periods, meditation proved to be an extremely helpful tool in coping with my situation, in terms of spiritual, mental, and physical health and well-being. I could personally verify the research that had been documented by various scientists in terms of the enormous potential of meditation in the health sector and for the coping process.[1,2,and 3]

By practicing meditation on the inner light and sound[4,5,and 6] as taught by Sant Rajinder Singh Ji, I experienced an increase in mental stability and harmony after each meditation sitting, accompanied by relaxation and calm, mentally and physically. Whenever tasks became overwhelming, a period of sitting in meditation helped me regain calm and stability.

It also helped me to become more aware of my body physically, as it became easier to get in touch with my paralyzed limbs through an inner sense of observing. I would describe it as an inner sense of being aware of energies in the body irrespective of whether nerve connections were intact or not. This inner sense of connection was awakened and strengthened by meditation. It helps me connect with my paralyzed limbs mentally, to feel energy sensations, and to create sympathy for the paralyzed body parts, which are sometimes neglected and almost forgotten by many individuals after a spinal cord injury followed by paralysis. I care and treat those body parts well, I am in touch with them, train them with electrostimulation and stretching daily and include them consciously in my individual body picture. I feel much more as a complete human being also physically despite the loss of motor control and senses, and meditation is helpful in this aspect.

Pain sensations were reduced through relaxation and stress reduction, both mentally and physically, through meditation.

In summary, I personally wish to point out that the spiritual way of looking at life was the first great help after the accident situation. To me, it is through the grace of God that I was able to experience this accident and everything that followed as a blessing without negative feelings or judgment. This grace is flowing through the unbounded spiritual presence and guidance of my spiritual Masters, Sant Darshan Singh Ji and Sant Rajinder Singh Ji, in my life.

In the process of rehabilitation and a handicapped life, this grace has continued. The love and care of Sant Rajinder Singh Ji always fills me with joy and gratitude at each moment of my life, even when things seemingly are difficult. Everything in my life has sense and meaning.

Life is not always easy, whether one faces physical challenges or other ones. With the teachings of the saints and all the blessings and support deriving from them, especially in my case the connection with Sant Darshan Singh Ji and Sant Rajinder Singh Ji, all is filled with meaning and trust that the best that could happen is actually happening. In our meetings, I feel charged with maximum love and support. Things are rather easy then. Even when we do not meet physically, these blessings continue and support my whole being. Everything is fine with the grace of God.

The process of meditation is a most valuable tool in regaining and keeping spiritual, mental, and physical health. It helps to recharge, to harmonize body and mind, and to widen the perspective for a spiritual vision of life.[7] It is a beautiful fact that in meditation one does not experience the limitations of the physical body. Meditation on inner light and sound is a peaceful, joyful experience, and I recommend it strongly to anyone who faces a physically limiting situation and is ready to try inner work to experience the benefits for himself or herself.

Harald M. Hoermann, M.S. (Biology) is a lecturer and scientist at Innsbruck Medical University, Austria. He is a seminar leader who facilitates the broadening of students' appreciation of individuals with handicaps and of life fulfillment despite a handicap. He teaches meditation techniques to medical students in the field of health promotion and stress management to people in high-level stress environments. His professional efforts are focused in active research on the role of meditation in a modern strategy of health promotion as well as counseling in stress management approaches. The health impact of meditation in daily life is his main research activity. In addition, he has a sports career as both an athlete and trainer, and after having had a sports accident more than twenty years ago is still competing as a hand-cyclist.

CHAPTER 15

MEDITATION AND HEALING PAIN

By James Harris Gruft, M.D., DABPM, FAAPMR

Meditation and Physical Pain

Persistent physical pain is multidimensional. Melzak and Casey describe three of pain's dimensions. There is the *sensory or noxious component* coming from the affected part that sends signals from our peripheral nerves to our brain. There is the *cognitive/evaluative component* of the pain: is it more intense, deeper, hotter, sharper, or more localized than the pain we had when we were six and we were hit in the stomach with a swing. Lastly, there is the *affective component* of the pain, where all the wrongs, all the unfairness ever dealt to us fans our pain like a blower in a huge medieval hearth.

Meditation both is and isn't the ultimate distraction technique. The word *distraction* comes from the word "tract" which means, "to draw (along)," and "dis" which means "away." Therefore, "distraction" means to draw away from—in this case—the pain. However, with meditation, we draw away from the pain not by escaping from it but by going through and beyond it. As one learns how to meditate, a wonderful calming experience arises that is soothing to the nerves, accompanied by a sweet sense of peace. Experiences like these help to minimize the suffering and the cognitive and affective dimensions of pain.

Pain, Suffering, and Darian

I once evaluated a man in his fifties who was in pain, whom I will call Darian. He had severe, chronic lower-back pain and was admitted into our pain-management program. He was taught and began practicing meditation. After engaging in this practice, he reported to me that while his pain could still be intense at times, it seldom hurt anymore. Sometimes he was able to shrug it off completely. On questioning him further, I discovered that what he really meant was that he continued to have pain but that there was no longer any suffering involved. The emotional turmoil that came with the pain, the suffering, was what had previously been so hard to bear; without this suffering, he could deal with his pain much more easily.

This process is often a gradual one, not as dramatic as Darian's case. However, the ability to reach this state is real. The calming and centering effects of meditation go a long way toward positively modifying our experience of pain. Recalling Melzak and Casey's 3-D model of pain, it appears that the cognitive/discriminative and the affective/motivational dimensions of the pain are most easily altered by meditation.[1] There may still be pain, but it is pain no longer aggravated by stress, tension, and the many wrongs we have suffered. A sense of healthy detachment develops as we meditate. This is not to be confused with dissociation, which is a form of escape. With healthy detachment, the pain has been processed and put in its proper context. By listening to the pain yet not succumbing to it, not letting it dominate our lives, pain becomes more manageable.

Meditation and Psychological Pain

Are we nothing more than the sum total of our body, feelings, and thoughts; or are we something besides that, beyond our likes and dislikes? Moreover, if our soul is something other than our thoughts and feelings, what function does it have?

Sant Rajinder Singh Ji Maharaj has described the outer expression of the soul as the attention.[2] Studies of the attention by scientists have verified that it is precognitive: it is present before actual thoughts are formed.[3] Because the attention occurs before thoughts, it should be possible to control which thoughts we have. But how many of us can do that? For most of us, our attention is in a weakened state and is incessantly pulled by external attractions or internal feelings. Consequently, we find ourselves obsessing over past experiences, dwelling on our pain, or being continuously distracted by nothing in particular. Joseph Chilton Pearce, author of *The Crack in the Cosmic Egg*, refers to this as "roof brain chatter."

Through the process of meditation and self-introspection, we can begin to experience ourselves as something beyond our likes and dislikes. We can become more attached to our self and less attached to the winds of time and their ever-changing panorama. Meditation strengthens our attention, which gives our soul more control over our thoughts and feelings; we are less overwhelmed by outer circumstances and by unpleasant experiences. We begin to realize that our life in the world is not our only reality; we see that our life also has a spiritual dimension.

What are the outward signs of people who have gained possession of their attention? They regularly take time away from the whirling barrage of activities that we call living in the twenty-first century, and focus their attention inside themselves in order to experience who they truly are. They are centered, and they maintain their equipoise, even amidst utter devastation.

With meditation, we can experience calmness. Psychological turmoil can be replaced by a peaceful sense of our selves. In addition, we may begin to experience a connection with the power that created all things. The more we contact that power, the more our attention will turn to our higher self.

Healing Our Pain through Spirituality and Meditation

Spirituality is appearing more frequently in medical literature. In a recent survey, measures of spirituality or religion were found in most of the major journals in 1 to 3 percent of their articles. In the medical journals in palliative medicine, 6.3 % had measures of spirituality or religion.[4] Why is spirituality expressed twice as frequently in the palliative-medicine literature? Palliative medicine is the branch of medicine concerned with relieving, not curing; it deals with people in chronic pain or at the end of their lives. These two conditions may lead people to explore the deepest aspects of their lives, which would include spirituality.

According to a recent Gallup poll, 95% of Americans believe in God or a higher power, with 85% indicating religious or spiritual beliefs are important in their lives.[5] Earlier polls showed that 43% stated they had been aware of, or influenced by, a presence or a power (whether or not they called it God) that was different from their everyday self.[6]

We may be healthy physically and psychologically, but if we believe our life has no meaning, we suffer from sickness of the soul. Under this cloud, we may move through our days but only skim the surface of our life. All the accouterments of the good life may be ours, even as we continuously anesthetize ourselves with distractions due to a hidden sense of emptiness. Our need to escape may lead to activities as useless as endlessly watching TV reruns, as profound as listening to a Beethoven string quartet, or as harmful as an addiction to alcohol or drugs. Regardless of our method of distraction, the purpose is the same: to escape from the pain caused by a lack of meaning in our life. Any painful reminder of something missing is pain. If we choose not to face this pain, it will be forced into the shadows, where it may emerge anytime in the form of utter despair or panic.

If we stop to think about it, the world is not a nurturing place. As we grow up, we are provided with innumerable distractions, which, together with our diversion-loving mind, keep us so engaged in the enjoyments and travails of the world that we seldom take the time to figure out what our life is all about. Under such circumstances, the rare wake-up call—the time when we suddenly realize with full force that we do not know what our purpose in life is—may hit us suddenly and threaten to overwhelm us. Unfortunately, rather than taking this realization further, most of us sweep this pain under the rug as fast as we can.

Sometimes, however, this profound experience shakes us enough to witness the deeper part of our being. One of the most profound events we can have is the death of someone we love. One fateful day, during my residency in physical medicine and rehabilitation at Columbia Presbyterian Hospital in Manhattan, the phone rang. It was my sister, sobbing, telling me that my father, who was in Spain vacationing with my mother, had suddenly died. The news was so sudden and shocking that it tore the fabric of my world apart.

At that point in my life, I saw what people in the East call *maya* (the illusion of the world). With blinding certainty, I realized that our entire culture was based on the illusion that we will live forever and that the goal of life was to live, drink, and be merry—or the modern equivalent: "whoever dies with the most toys wins." As a result of that experience, I sought a deeper meaning in my life. Many enticements of the world lost their power over me.

As much as we may acknowledge that we won't live forever, how many of us truly believe that? We prefer to live under the spell of false immortality rather than face the truth, a condition I call collective denial. Ignoring the implications of our mortality, we all believe that if we read enough good books, watch enough good movies, go on enough great vacations, make enough money, use enough antiaging creams or pills, have enough face-lifts or surgical tucks, exercise enough, eat enough good food, surround ourselves with enough beauty, and have enough of our fantasies come true, we will somehow escape the inevitability of old age and death. If that isn't illusion, what is?

When a person realizes his or her complete helplessness and in humility cries out to God for help, that is a cry of the soul. According to Sant Rajinder Singh Ji, "By true prayer and a sincere longing, God listens to our cries."[7] After that cry has escaped from our heart and flown to the heavens, we can do nothing but wait. Some spiritual traditions assert that if we sincerely cry out from the depths of our soul to the Creator, God will respond by bringing us to someone who can teach us how to contact our deeper, inner self. Then, like a primitive forest dweller being shown how to kneel before a pond, we may see our face for the first time. Quieting our mind and withdrawing our attention from the outer world is the beginning of seeing our true face, our inner self. This act of gazing into the pool, far from being an act of narcissism, is one that arises out of an authentic love for our soul. It is the ultimate act of charity to ourselves, allowing us to have a break from our mind, which is always seeking to drag us here and there. This process of looking within, called prayer with attention or meditation, aids us in discovering our spiritual nature—a nature beyond fears and mundane concerns, beyond our petty likes and dislikes. And it must be done alone.

Our loneliness is most keenly felt in the spaces between our distractions: in between our work, our TV shows, our romantic life, and our addictions. It fills in the gaps between our adventures with alcohol, cigarettes, or drugs, rising from the shadows whenever we find ourselves alone. It looms over our heads, ready to pounce *when we have nothing to do.*

The remarkable thing is that if we don't try to run away when the pain appears, and instead just look at it and wait there silently and do nothing—once this pain has finished trying to overwhelm us, it will begin to speak. The first words it usually utters are, "What are you doing with your life?" Where on earth are these words coming from?

There is a power we can harness that can help us achieve mental peace and develop a strong sense of self, strong enough to stand up for our principles and not lose out to our addictions.

It is the power that comes from being alone.

Being utterly alone may be terrifying for someone who has never experienced it. It means isolating ourselves from anything that can pull our attention outside, into the world. This is different from distracting ourselves from our pain. We do not try to get away from the pain; we face it. In the practice of Jyoti Meditation, in which we are essentially alone, we are not focusing on our breathing; we are making a conscious effort to eliminate influences, including those of our body.

It takes great courage to be essentially alone, to do what is called meditation. Meditation, though associated with most religions, is not in and of itself a religious practice. It is simply a tool for deepening our connection with ourselves and our higher power. We may choose to meditate whether we are theists or atheists. Many years ago, when I started practicing meditation, I must admit that there were times I felt miserable sitting alone, cut off from others. I wondered why I was taking precious time away from my busy life when it seemed that all I got out of it was more pain than when I started. Part of me screamed to be "out there"—running around, working, creating, meeting people—in short, conquering the world. However, a deeper, quieter part of me felt the need to develop an inner life. I had failed to find the meaning of life "out there" and was barely keeping the despair of meaninglessness from engulfing me. I maintained it with the guidance and encouragement of two Masters of meditation. Since then I have changed. I have become more centered, possessing a deeper inner life. Looking back, I believe it was one of the most courageous things I have ever done.

Sant Rajinder Singh Ji describes a simple meditation process, called Jyoti Meditation, in his book, *Inner and Outer Peace through Meditation*. He asks that we close our eyes and, fully awake—in a quiet place where we will not be distracted, where we won't be disturbed—we focus our attention in front of us and begin to meditate. It is here, finally, that we are alone. To keep our mind from distracting us with mundane or seemingly profound thoughts, which are the last formidable distractions, we keep the mind busy by repeating any Name for the higher power or virtue that we feel comfortable with. With the mind engaged so it will not bother us, we sit, watch, and wait. For what? For whatever we receive. It is an effective meditation technique that I follow and encourage my patients with chronic pain to practice. (See the last chapter for the instructions for the Jyoti Meditation technique, the introductory form of meditation, given by Sant Rajinder Singh Ji Maharaj.)

As I said, being alone takes courage. The process of stopping the inner chatter of our mind also takes practice and patience. In the face of many distractions, lack of sensory stimulation can seem daunting.

If we wish to face our pain we must heroically make a stand, and we must do it alone. What are heroes? They are people who live up to their principles, regardless of the circumstances. Many of us secretly wish to be heroes, but exactly how are they made? Is it only when the dragon comes out of its lair that the hero's might is tested? No. A real hero does not need fantastical enemies. One who can successfully face the major and minor catastrophes of the day is a hero.

Joseph Campbell, the great mythologist, closes his masterpiece, *The Hero with a Thousand Faces*, by considering the relationship between meditation and the hero.

"The preliminary meditations of the aspirant detach his mind and sentiments from the accidents of life and drive him to the core. 'I am not that, not that,' he meditates: 'not my mother or son who has just died; my body, which is ill or aging . . . I am not my mind; not my power of intuition.' By such meditations he is driven to his own profundity and breaks through, at last, to unfathomable realizations .... The aim is not to see, but to

203

realize that one is, that essence .... Wherever the hero may wander, whatever he may do, he is ever in the presence of his own essence—for he has the perfected eye to see."[8]

Therefore, the true act of the hero is not connected to his or her actions against tyranny, hypocrisy, or evil. That which marks the heroic is the act of being alone. For it is this act, hidden from all eyes, filled with inexplicable pains and frustrations, which seeks to invoke grace and enables one to rise to another level of consciousness. Thus is the heart of the hero opened. One hopes that it may be an experience blessed with divine revelation, but there can be no expectations. The hero must wait; whatever is meant to come will come.

The act of being alone constitutes the unseen part of the hero's life, unknown to observers of her or his great feats of courage, which are hidden from her or his biographers. During the process of meditation, of being alone, a deeper sense of one's self develops. It is the process of looking inside. Through meditation, we withdraw our attention from the outside and focus it within, to a place beyond our emotions and thoughts. Instead of its usual tendency to go to the outer attractions or into feelings or thoughts, the attention is turned inside to realize our third aspect: the soul.

In many ways, spiritual pain is the final frontier. What is our endpoint but finding out who we are, what we are doing with our life, and where we are going after our physical existence ceases? Can such a pain ever be ameliorated? The answer is tied to being essentially alone, where we enter into deep silence and engage in prayer-with-attention (a term for meditation). Meditation is a way to connect with our deeper self and the higher power. The deeper we are able to connect, the less our separation and the more we gain a powerful source of strength within.

James H. Gruft, M.D., DABPM, FAAPMR, and Medical Director is board-certified in Physical Medicine & Rehabilitation and Pain Medicine. He served as medical director of Marianjoy Rehabilitation Hospital's Comprehensive Pain Management Program in Chicagoland for more than 14 years. Presently, he is assistant professor at Rush University Medical Center Department of Physical Medicine and Rehabilitation, teaching resident physicians the art and science of pain medicine.

A nationally recognized doctor & author, Dr. James Gruft is also the founder of the pain management and lifestyle medicine health center From Pain to Wellness. He is the author of a popular book, *From Pain to Wellness*, on pain management.

Dr. Gruft has been nationally recognized by his peers as a "Best Doctor" for the years 2002 to present, and is respected by physicians across the country as "one of the premier pain specialists practicing today."

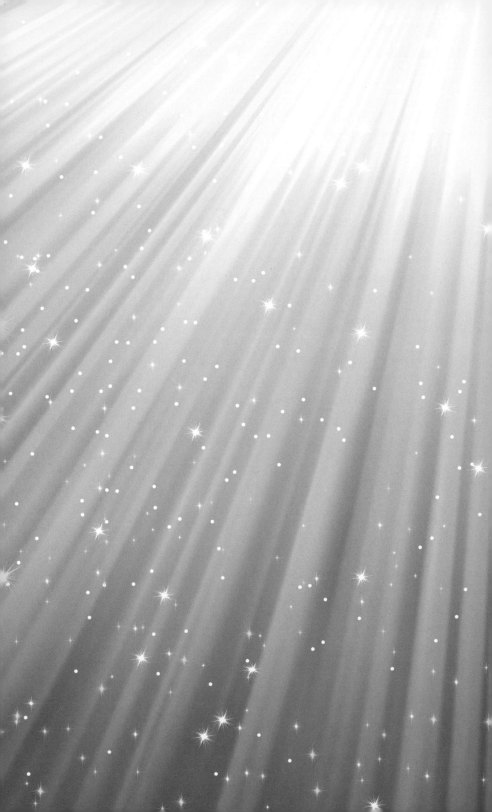

PART 7

Meditation Technique

CHAPTER 16:

JYOTI MEDITATION INSTRUCTIONS

by Sant Rajinder Singh Ji Maharaj

Jyoti Meditation (light meditation) is an introductory practice we can try on our own. To meditate, we sit in a comfortable pose, most convenient to us, in which we can sit still for the longest possible time. While meditating, we do not hold hands or touch anyone else, as any movement brings our attention back down into the body, distracting us from concentration on the seat of the soul, also called the third eye, single eye, *shiv netra*, *divya chakshu*, *ajna* or *aggya chakra*, tenth door, or *daswan dwar* (located between and behind the two eyebrows).

We close our eyes, gently, as we do when we go to sleep, but we remain wide awake. Closing our eyes keeps us from being distracted by the outer sights of the physical world. With closed eyes, we focus our attention in front of us. We do not put pressure on our eyes. We also do not raise our eyes upwards towards the direction of the eyebrows as that puts pressure on our eyes and forehead and can result in a headache. Rather, we keep our eyes focused gently in front of us and look into the middle of what appears within. We keep gazing horizontally, focusing about eight to ten inches in front of us with closed eyes.

We look lovingly into the middle of what appears in front of us. We may at first see either darkness or light, sparks of light, pinpoints of light, flashes of light, circles of light, or light of any color, such as red, orange, yellow, blue, green, purple, violet, white, or golden color. We should continue gazing into the middle of what appears. We may see inner vistas such as an inner sky, clouds, stars, a moon, or a sun.

While looking into the middle of what appears, we may notice that our mind sends thoughts that distract us from gazing within. We may find that we cannot silence our mind to continue meditating. To help keep our mind from distracting us, we can mentally and silently repeat any Name of God with which we feel comfortable. This repetition should go on mentally, and not aloud, as we continue to gaze. By gazing deeper into the middle of the light, we can tap into the spiritual treasures within and enjoy profound peace, bliss, and happiness unlike any we have found in this world. Divine love engulfs and fulfills us. The beauty of meditation is that this joy remains with us even after we resume our daily activities.

References and End Notes

Chapter 1: Meditation as Medication for the Soul, by Sant Rajinder Singh Ji Maharaj

[1] Craven, Dr. John L. (1989), Meditation and Psychotherapy, Canadian *Journal of Psychiatry*, Vol. 34, October 1989, pp. 648-53.

[2] Kutz, MD, Ilan, *et al.* (1985), Meditation and Psychotherapy, *American Journal of Psychiatry*, Vol. 142, January 1985, pp. 1-8.

Chapter 2: Meditation: 25 Years Experience in Primary Care Medicine, by Matthew Raider, M.D.

[1] Wallace, R. K. & Benson, H. (1972). The physiology of meditation. *Sci. Amer,* 262(2):84-90.

[2] Bagchi, B. K. & Wenger, M. A. (1957). Electrophysiological correlates of some yogi exercises. *Electroencephaologr. Clin. Neurophysiol,* (Suppl)7:132-149.

[3] Dillbeck, M. C. & Orme-Johnson, D. W. (1987). Psychological differences between transcendental meditation and rest. *Am. Psychol,* 42:879-881.

[4] Werner, O., Wallace, R. K., Charles, B., Janssen, G., & Chalmers, R. (1989). Endocrine balance and the TM-Sidhi programme. Collected papers (Vol 2). Rheinweiler, Germany: MERU Press.

[5] Glaser, J. L., Brind, J. L., Vogelman, J. H., et.al. (1991). Elevated serum dehydroepiandrosterone sulfate levels in practitioners of

the transcendental meditation and TM-Sidhi programs. *Journal of Behavioral Medicine,* 15:327-341.

[6] Das, N. N., (1957). Fastaut, H. Variations de L'Activite Electrique du Cerveau du Coeur et des Muscles quelletiques au Cours de la meditation et de l'extase yogique. *Electroencephologr. Clin. Neurophysiol,* 6(Suppl.):211-219.

[7] Orme-Johnson, D. W., & Haynes, C. T. (1981). EEG phase coherence, pure consciousness, creativity and TM-Sidhi experiences. *Int. J. Neurosci,* 13:211-217.

[8] Benson, H., & Wallace, R. K. (1972). Decreased blood pressure in hypertensive subjects who practiced meditation. *Circulation,* 45-46(Suppl.):516(a).

[9] Schneider, R. H., Alexander, C. N., Staggers, F., et. al. (2005). Long-term effects of stress reduction on mortality in persons> or=55 years of age with systemic hypertension. *Am. Journal Cardiology,* 95(9):1060-1064.

[10] Zamarra, J. W., Schneider, R. H., Besseghini, I., Robinson, D. K., & Salerno, J. W. (1996). Usefulness of the transcendental meditation program in the treatment of patients with coronary artery disease. *Am Journal of Cardiology,* 77(10):867-870.

[11] Curiati, J. A., Bocchi, E., Freire, J. O., Arantes, A. C., et. al. (2005). Meditation reduces sympathetic activation and improves the quality of life in elderly patients with optimally treated heart failure: a prospective randomized study, *Journal of Alt. & Comp. Med,* 11(3):465-472.

[12] Kaplan, K. H., Goldenberg, D. L., & Galvin-Nadeau, M. (1993). The impact of a meditation-based stress reduction program on fibromyalgia. *Gen. Hosp. Psych,* 15:284-289.

[13] Speigel, D. (1989). Effect of psycho-social treatment of patients with metastatic breast cancer. *Lancet,* 2:888-891, 1989

[14] Relman, A. (1988). Effectiveness of relaxation of visualization techniques as an adjunct to phototherapy of psoriasis. *Journal Am. Acad. Dermatol,* 19:572-573.

[15] Bujatti, M., & Riederer, P. (1976). Serotonin, noradrenaline, and dopamine metabolites in the transcendental meditation technique. *Journal Neural Transm,* 39:257-267.

[16] Wilson, R. S., Barnes, L. L., Bennett, D. A., Y Li, & Bienes, J. L. (2005). Proneness to psychological distress and the risk of Alzheimer's disease in a biracial community. *Neurology,* 64:380-382.

[17] Kim, D. H., Moon, Y. S., Kim, H. S., et. al. (2005). Effect of Zen meditation on serum nitric oxide activity and lipid peroxidation. *Progress in Neuro-psych. & Bio. Psych.* 29(2):327-331.

[18] Penfield, W. (1975). *The Mystery of the Mind.* Princeton, New Jersey: Princeton University Press.

Chapter 3: Cancer: How Meditation Can Provide a Lifeline, by Saraswati Sukamar, Ph.D., Professor of Oncology, Breast Cancer Program, Johns Hopkins School of Medicine, Baltimore, MD

[1] Jemal, A., Bray, F., Center, M.M., Ferlay, J., Ward, E., & Forman, D.. Global cancer statistics. CA Cancer J Clin. 2011 Mar-Apr;61(2):69-90. *PubMed* PMID: 212968551:

[2] DeSantis, C., Siege, I.R., Bandi, P., & Jemal, A. Breast cancer statistics, 2011. CA Cancer J Clin. 2011 Nov-Dec;61(6):409-18. doi: 10.3322/caac.20134. *Epub* 2011 Oct Review. PubMed PMID: 21969133.

[3] Hede, K. Supportive care: large studies ease yoga, exercise into mainstream oncology. J Natl Cancer Inst. 2011 Jan 5;103(1):11-2. *Epub* 2010 Dec 17. *PubMed* PMID: 21169537.

[4] Matchim, Y., Armer, J.M., Stewart, BR. Mindfulness-based stress reduction among breast cancer survivors: a literature review and discussion. *Oncol Nurs Forum.* 2011 Mar;38(2):E61-71. Review. PubMed PMID: 21356643.

[5] Chopra, D., Medicine's Great Divide- the view from the alternative side, *Virtual Mentor.* **June 2011,** Volume 13, Number 6: 394-398.

Chapter 4: Meditation in the Modern World, by Kunwarjit Singh Duggal, M.D.

[1] Geary, C. & Rosenthal, S.L. (2011). Sustained impact of MBSR on stress, well-being, and daily spiritual experiences for 1 year in academic health care employees. *Journal of Alternative and Complementary Medicine*, Vol. 17, October 2011, pp. 939-44.

[2] Cutshall, S.M., Wentworth, L.J., Wahner-Roedler, D.L., Vincent, A., Schmidt, J.E., Loehrer, L.L., Cha, S.S. & Bauer, B.A. (2011). Evaluation of a biofeedback-assisted meditation program as a stress management tool for hospital nurses: a pilot study. *Explore*, Vol. 7, March-April 2011, pp. 110-2.

[3] Warnecke, E., Quinn, S., Ogden, K., Towle, N. & Nelson, M.R. (2011). A randomized controlled trial of the effects of mindfulness practice on medical student stress levels. *Medical Education*, Vol. 45, April 2011, pp. 381-8.

[4] Malinski, V.M. & Todaro-Franceschi, V. (2011). Exploring co-meditation as a means of reducing anxiety and facilitating relaxation in a nursing school setting. *Journal of Holistic Nursing*, Vol. 29, December 2011, pp. 242-8.

[5] Zeidan, F., Martucci, K.T., Kraft, R.A., Gordon, N.S., McHaffie, J.G. & Coghill, R.C. (2011). Brain mechanisms supporting the modulation of pain by mindfulness meditation. *The Journal of Neuroscience*, Vol. 31, April 2011, pp. 5540-8.

[6] Choi, K.E., Rampp, T., Saha, F.J., Dobos, G.J. & Musial F. (2011) m Pain modulation by meditation and electroacupuncture in experimental submaximum effort tourniquet technique. *Explore*, Vol. 7, July-August 2011, pp. 239-45.

[7] Schmidt, S., Srossman, P., Schwarzer, B., Jena, S., Naumann, J. & Walach, H. (2011). Treating fibromyalgia with mindfulness-based stress reduction: results from a 3-armed randomized controlled trial, *Pain*, Vol. 152, February 2011, pp. 361-9.

[8] Hennard, J. (2011). A protocol and pilot study for managing fibromyalgia with yoga and meditation. *International Journal of Yoga Therapy*. Vol. 21, 2011, pp. 109-21.

[9] Fox, S.D., Flynn, E. & Allen, R.H. (2011). Mindfulness meditation for women with chronic pelvic pain: a pilot study. *Journal of Reproductive Medicine*. Vol. 56, March-April 2011, pp. 158-62.

[10] Teixeira, E. (2010). The effect of mindfulness meditation on painful diabetic peripheral neuropathy in adults older than 50 years. *Holistic Nursing Practice*. Vol. 24, September-October 2010, pp. 277-83.

[11] Radi, D.I., Vieten, C., Michel, L. & Delorme, A. (2011). Electrocortical activity prior to unpredictable stimuli in meditators and nonmeditators. *Explore*. Vol. 7, September-October 2011, pp. 286-99.

[12] Travis, F. (2011). Comparison of coherence, amplitude, and eLORETA patterns during transcendental Meditation and TM-Sidhi practice. *International Journal of Psychophysiology*. Vol. 81, September 2011, pp. 198-202.

[13] Engstrom, M., Pihlsgard, J., Lundberg, P., & Soderfeldt, B. (2010). Functional magnetic resonance imaging of hippocampal activation during silent mantra meditation. *Journal of Alternative and Complementary Medicine*. Vol. 16, December 2010, pp. 1253-8.

[14] Moss, A.S., Wintering, N., Roggenkamp, H, Khalsa, D.S., Waldman, M.R., Monti, D. & Newberg, A.B. (2012). Effects of an 8-week meditation program on mood and anxiety in patients with memory loss. *Journal of Alternative and Complementary Medicine*. Vol. 18, January 2012, pp. 48-53.

[15] Newberg, A.B., Wintering, N., Khalsa, D.S., Roggenkamp, H. & Waldman, M.R. (2010). Meditation effects on cognitive function and cerebral blood flow in subjects with memory loss: a preliminary study. *Journal of Alzheimer's Disease*. Vol. 20, 2010, pp. 517-26.

[16] Zeidan, F., Johnson, S.K., Diamond, B.J., David, Z. & Goolkasian, P. (2010). Mindfulness meditation improves cognition: evidence of brief mental training. *Consciousness and Cognition*. Vol. 19, June 2010, pp. 597-605.

Chapter 5: Meditation for Emotional Wellness, by Mark E. Young, Ph.D.

Aftanas, L., & Golosheykin, S. (2005). Impact of regular meditation practice on EEG activity at rest and during evoked negative emotions. *International Journal of Neuroscience, 115*(6), 893-909.

Benson, H., & Stark, M. (1996). *Timeless healing: The power and biology of belief.* New York: Scribner.

Folkman, S., & Lazarus, R. S. (1980). An analysis of coping in a middle-aged community sample. *Journal of Health and Social Behavior, 21,* 219-239.

Goleman, D. (1995). *Emotional intelligence.* New York: Bantam.

Goleman, D., & Schwartz, G. (1976). Meditation as an intervention in stress reactivity. *Journal of Consulting and Clinical Psychology, 44*(3), 456-466.

Lane, J., Seskevich, J., & Pieper, C. (2007). Brief meditation training can improve perceived stress and negative mood. *Alternative Therapies in Health & Medicine, 13*(1), 38-44.

Smith, W. P., Compton, W.C., & Beryl, W. (1995). Meditation as an adjunct to a happiness enhancement program. *Journal of Clinical Psychology, 51,* 260-273.

Wachholtz, A., & Pargament, K. (2005). Is spirituality a critical Ingredient of meditation? Comparing the effects of spiritual meditation, secular meditation, and relaxation on spiritual, psychological, cardiac, and pain outcomes. *Journal of Behavioral Medicine, 28*(4), 369-384.

Chapter 6: The Creative Factor in Spirituality and Health, by Debbie Purdy, M.A.A.T

Cassou, M. (2001). *Point Zero.* New York: Tarcher/Putman.

Cassou, M., & Cubley, S. (1995). *Life, Paint and Passion.* New York: Tarcher/Putnam.

Csikszentmihalyi, M. (1990). *Flow.* New York: Harper Row.

Ganin, B. (1999). *Art and Healing*. New York: Three Rivers Press.

Gardner, H. (1982). *Art, Mind and Brain*. New York: Basic Books.

McNiff, S. (1992). *Art as Medicine*. Boston: Shambala Publications.
Samuels, M. & Rockwood–Lane, M. (1998). *Creative Healing*. New York: Harper Collins.

Chapter 7: Spirituality and Mental Health, by John McGrew, Ph.D.

Levin, J. (2001). God, Faith, and Health: Exploring the Spirituality - Healing Connection. New York: John Wiley & Sons.

Freud, S. (1989). *The Future of an Illusion*. (first published in 1927). New York: W. W. Norton & Company.

Faith and Healing: Can spirituality promote health? Time Magazine, June 24, 1996

Gallup Poll Social Series: Values and Beliefs, May 8-11, 2008

Koenig, H.G., McCullough, M.E., & Larson, D.B. (editors). (2001). *Handbook of Religion and Health*. New York: Oxford University Press.
Benor, D.J. (2001). *Spiritual Healing: Scientific Validation of a Healing Revolution*. Southfield, MI: Vision Publications.

Chapter 8: FAQs on Mental Health and Spirituality, by Marshall O. Zaslove, M.D.

[1] Kusler, R. C., & Chu, W. T. (2005). Prevalence, Severity, and Comorbidity of 12-Month DSM-IV Disorders in the National Comorbidity Survey Replication. *Arch Gen Psychiatry*, 62:617-627.

[2] Sanson, R. A., & Khatain, K. (1990). The Role of Religion in Psychiatric Training. *Academic Psychiatry*, 14: 34-38.

[3] Gotlib, I. H., & Hammen, C. L. (2010). *Handbook of Depression, Second Edition*. New York: Guilford, p. 510.

[4] Levin, J. S., & Larson D. B. (1997). Religion and Spirituality in Medicine: Research and Education. *JAMA*, 278:792-793.

[5] Gartner, J., & Larson, D. B. (1991). Religious Commitment and Mental Health. *Psychology and Theology*, 19:6-25.

[6] Shafranske, E.P. (2000). Religious Involvement and Professional Practices of Psychiatrists. *Psychiatric Annals*, 30:525-532.

[7] Fortney, L. (2010). Meditation in Medical Practice: A Review of the Evidence and Practice. *Primary Care*, 37:1, 81-90.

[8] Selye, H. (1978). *The Stress of Life*. New York: McGraw Hill.

[9] Benson, H. & Klipper, M. (1976), *The Relaxation Response*. New York: Harper Torch.

[10] Moody, R. A. *Life After Life*. (2001). New York: Harper One.

Chapter 9: Meditation: Finding Our Balance, by Rimjhim Duggal Stephens, M.B.B.S.

[1] Lagopoulos et al. (2009) Increased Theta and Alpha EEG Activity during Nondirective Meditation. *The Journal of Alternative and Complementary Medicine*, 2009; 15 (11): 1187 doi: 10.1089/acm.2009.0113

[2] Lavretsky, H., Epel, E.S., Siddarth, P., Nazarian, N., Cyr, N.S., Khalsa, D.S., Lin. J., Blackburn, E., & Irwin, M.R. (2012). A Pilot Study of Yogic Meditation for Family Dementia Caregivers with Depressive Symptoms: Effects on Mental Health, Cognition, and Telomerase Activity. *Int J Geriatr Psychiatry.* 2012. Mar 11. doi: 10.1002/gps.3790

[3] Chaterji, R., Tractenberg, R.E., Amri, H., Lumpkin, M., Amorosi, S.B., & Haramati, A. (2007) A large-sample survey of first- and second-year medical student attitudes toward complementary and alternative medicine in the curriculum and in practice. *Altern Ther Health Med.* 2007. Jan-Feb; 13(1): 30-5.

[4] Ishak, W.W., Lederer, S., Mandili, C., Nikravesh, R., Seligman, L., Vasa, M., Ogunyemi, D., & Bernstein, C.A. (2009). Burnout during residency training: a literature review. *J Grad Med Educ.* 2009. Dec;1(2):.236-42.

[5] Paul, G., Elam, B., & Verhulst, S.J. (2007). A longitudinal study of students' perceptions of using deep breathing meditation to reduce testing stresses. *Teach Learn Med*. 2007. Summer;.19(3):.287-92.

Chapter 10: Meditation and Spirituality: A Homeopath's Perspective, by Tim Fior, M.D., D.Ht.

[1] Homeopathy is a 200 year old system of healing developed by a physician, Samuel Hahnemann, in Germany. The basic principle is the law of similars or that like cures like. Also, in homeopathy generally infinitesimally diluted medicines are used one at a time. For this reason, homeopathic medicines are much safer than conventional and even herbal medicines.

[2] WHO is the World Health Organization. Health is defined on their website (http://www.who.int/about/definition/en/) as "a state of complete physical, mental and social well-being and not merely the absence of disease or infirmity.
The correct bibliographic citation for the definition is:
Preamble to the Constitution of the World Health Organization as adopted by the International Health Conference, New York, 19-22 June 1946; signed on 22 July 1946 by the representatives of 61 States (Official Records of the World Health Organization, no. 2, p. 100) and entered into force on 7 April 1948.
The Definition has not been amended since 1948."

[3] Laszlo, Ervin. *The Whispering Pond*. Element, Rockport Massachusetts, 1996, p.108-110.

[4] Ibid.

[5] Bell, I. R., Lewis, D. A. I., Schwartz, G. E., Lewis, S. E., Caspi, O., Scott, A., Brooks, A. J. and Baldwin, C. M. (2004). Electroencephalographic
cordance patterns distinguish exceptional clinical responders with
fibromyalgia to individualized homeopathic medicines. *J Alternative & Complementary Medicine* 10, 285-299.

[6] Homeopathic medicines above 12C potency are so highly diluted (and succussed or shaken at each dilution) that the active

ingredient has been diluted out. Somehow they retain some information (possibly some form of electromagnetic signature or remnant nanoparticles) from the original active ingredient that is then able to react with someone who is highly sensitive to this particular information.

[7] Starfield, Barbara. Is US health Really the Best in the World? *JAMA*, July 26, 2000; Vol 284, no. 4, p. 483-485.

[8] Jonas, Wayne. A critical Overview of Homeopathy. *Ann Intern Med*. 2003;138:393-399.

[9] These guideposts in homeopathy are called Hering's rule, which states that symptoms tend to disappear in the reverse order of appearance (i.e. most recent first), from above downwards, from inside to outside, and from more important to less important organ. Of course, there are exceptions to this rule, but the point is that this is a way to tell if things are headed in the right direction.

[10] Esp. (2007b). *Empowering your Soul through Meditation*. Lisle, Illinois: Radiance Publishers.

[11] Notably mindfulness meditation in the Zen Buddhist tradition, and Transcendental Meditation.

[12] Benson, Herbert. *The Relaxation Response*. 1975. Harper Collins, New York.

[13] They noted an increase in alpha wave (7.5 to 13 cycles per second) activity which is slower than the normal beta brain wave (> or = 14 cycles per second) activity of the waking state. However, subsequent research has showed that meditation's effects on EEG patterns are much more complex than this simple generalization.

[14] These include positron emission tomography (PET), single photon emission computed tomography (SPECT), and functional magnetic resonance imaging (fMRI).

[15] Newberg, A.B. The neural basis of the complex mental task of meditation: neurotransmitter and neurochemical considerations. *Medical Hypotheses* (2003) 61(2), 282-291.

[16] GABA or gamma amino butyric acid is an inhibitory neurotransmitter produced in many regions of the Central Nervous System. An increase in its level would mean that fewer distracting outside stimuli would be processed, thus enhancing the sense of focus.

[17] Melatonin is a hormone produced in the pineal gland, which regulates sleep and declines with age. Serotonin is the neurotransmitter which Selective Serotonin Reuptake Inhibitors (SSRIs) like Prozac increase in the brain to overcome depression.

[18] Shapiro, S. An analysis of Recent Meditation Research and Suggestions for Future Directions. *Humanistic Psychologist*, 31, Spring and Summer 2003, p. 89.

[19] Morse, Melvin. *Transformed by the Light.* Ivy Books, New York, 1992.

Chapter 11: Chiropractic and Meditation: From Healing to Wholeness, by Alan R. Post, D.C.

[1] Breenan et al. (1991). Enhanced Phagocytic Cell Respiratory Bursts Induced by Spinal Manipulation. *Journal of Manipulative Therapeutic 199 14(7) 399-407*

[2] Chopra, D. (1989). *Quantum Healing: Exploring The Frontiers of Mind Body Medicine.* New York, USA: Bantam Books

[3] Singh, Darshan. (1982). *Spiritual Awakening.* Naperville, Illinois: SK Publications.

[4] Singh, Kirpal. (1967). *Godman.* Naperville, Illinois: SK Publications.

Chapter 12: Neurotheology: The Brain and the Science of
Meditation, by Louis A. Ritz, Ph.D.

Barnes, P. M., Bloom, B. & Nahin, R. L. 2008. *Complementary and
Alternative Medicine Use Among Adults and Children: United States,
2007.* National Health Statistics Reports. Number 12.

Beauregard, M. & O'Leary, D. (2007). *The Spiritual Brain: A
Neuroscientist's Case for the Existence of the Soul.* New York:
HarperCollins.

Beauregard, M. & Paquette, V. (2006). Neural Correlates of a
Mystical Experience in Carmelite Nuns. *Neurosci. Letters.* 405, 186-
190.

Beauregard, M. & Paquette, V. (2008). EEG Activity in Carmelite
Nuns during a Mystical Experience. *Neurosci. Letters.* 444, 1-4.

Begley, S. (2007). *Train Your Mind, Change your Brain: How a New
Science Reveals Our Extraordinary Potential to Transform Ourselves.*
New York: Ballantine Books.

Davidson, R. J. (2004). Well-being and affective style: neural
substrates and biobehavioural correlates. *Phil. Trans. R. Soc. Lond.
B.* 359: 1395-1411.

George, M. S. et al. (2010). Daily Left Prefrontal Transcranial
Magnetic Stimulation Therapy for Major Depressive Disorder: A
Sham-Controlled Randomized Trial. *Arch Gen Psychiatry.* 67:507-
516.

Holzel, B. K. et al. (2010). Mindfulness Meditation leads to
Increases in Regional Brain Gray Matter Density. *Psychiatry
Research: Neuroimaging.* 191: 36-43.

Kabat-Zinn, J. (2005). *Wherever You Go, There You Are: Mindfulness
Meditation in Everyday Life.* New York: Hyperion Books.

Lazar, S. W. et al. (2005). Meditation Experience is Associated with
Increased Cortical Thickness. *Neuroreport.* 16(17): 1893-1897.

Levin, J. (2002). *God, Faith, and Health: Exploring the Spirituality-Healing Connection*. New York: Wiley Press.

Lutz, A., Slagter, H. A., Dunne, J. D. & Davidson, R.J. (2008). Attention regulation and monitoring in meditation. *Trends in Cognitive Sciences*. 12 (4): 163-169.

Moody, R. (1976). *Life After Life*. Atlanta: Mockingbird Books.

Nadeau, S., Ferguson, T. S., Ritz, L. A., et.al. 2004. *Medical Neuroscience*. Philadelphia: Elsevier Press.

Nepo, M. (2006). *Unlearning Back to God: Essays on Inwardness, 1985-2005*. New York: Khaniqahi Nimatullahi Publications

Newberg, A. & D'Aquili, E. (2002). *Why God Won't Go Away: Brain Science and the Biology of Belief*. New York: Ballantine Books

Rubia, K. (2009). The Neurobiology of Meditation and its Clinical Effectiveness in Psychiatric Disorders. *Biological Psychology*. 82: 1-11.

Santorelli, S. (2000). *Heal Thy Self: Lessons on Mindfulness in Medicine*. New York: Three Rivers' Press.

Saver, J. L. & Rabin, J. (1997). The Neural Substrates of Religious Experience. *J. Neuropsych. Clin. Neurosciences*. 9: 498-510.

Singh, Darshan. 1978. *Secret of Secrets*. Naperville, Illinois: SK Publications.

Singh, Rajinder. (2005). *Silken Thread of the Divine*. Naperville, Illinois: SK Publications.

Singh, Rajinder. (2007a). *Inner and Outer Peace through Meditation*. Lisle, Illinois: Radiance Publishers.

Singh, Rajinder. (2007b). *Empowering Your Soul through Meditation*. Lisle, Illinois: Radiance Publishers.

Singh, Rajinder. (2011). *Spark of the Divine*. Lisle, Illinois: Radiance Publishers.

Slagter, H. A., Davidson, R. J. & Lutz, A. (2011). Mental Training as a Tool in the Neuro-scientific Study of Brain and Cognitive Plasticity. *Frontiers in Human Neuroscience.* 5: 1-12.

Tindle, H. A., Davis, R. B., Phillips, R. S., & Eisenberg, D. M. (2005). Trends in Use of Complementary and Alternative Medicine by U.S. Adults: 1997-2002. *Altern. Ther. Health Med.* Jan-Feb; 11(1):42-9.

Wallace, R. K. (1971). The Physiological Effects of Transcendental Meditation: A Proposed Fourth Major State of Consciousness. Doctoral Dissertation. University of California, Los Angeles.

Wallace, R. K., & Benson, H. (1972). The Physiology of Meditation. *Scientific American.* 226 (2): 84-90.

Walsh, R. (2000). *Essential Spirituality: The 7 Central Practices to Awaken Heart and Mind.* New York: Wiley Press.

Chapter 13: Reducing Stress-Related Ailments in Learners for Peak Performance, by Ricki Linksman, M.Ed.

[1] Beecham. John. (2009) "Study: Stress hits graduate students particularly hard: Survey finds many feel hopeless, consider suicide." *Daily Nebraskan*, March 9, 2009.

[2] Thomas, Caroline Bedell, MD and Murphy, Edmond. A, MD, Department of Medicine, The Johns Hopkins University School of Medicine, Baltimore, MD, (Sept. 5, 1958). "Further studies on cholesterol levels in the Johns Hopkins medical students: The effect of stress at examinations." *Journal of Chronic Disease*, December 1958. Vol. 8, Issue 6, pages 661-668.

[3] National Health Ministries. (2004) "Stress and the College Student." *PC (USA).* 7.2004 / Rev. 2. 2006.

[4] Ibid.

[5] Ibid.

[6] John Tung Foundation study. (2004) "Depression among Adolescents in Taipei Area."

[7] Kai-Wen, Cheng. Kaohsiung Hospitality College (2004) "A study of stress sources among college students." Taiwan: Journal of Academic and Business Ethics: p.1.

[8] Linksman, Ricki. (2001). *How to Learn Anything Quickly*. New York. Barnes and Noble.

[9] Singh, Rajinder. (2005) *Silken Thread of the Divine: Education for a Peaceful World*. Naperville, Illinois: SK Publications, p. 103.

[10] Pascual-Leone, Alvaro, Armedi, Amir, Fregni, Felipe, and Merabet, Lotfi B. (2005). "The Plastic Human Brain Cortex." Boston: Harvard College: Annu. Rev. Neurosci. 2005. 28:377-401.

[11] Tan, Yi-Yuan; Lu, Qilin; Geng, Siujuan; Stein, Eliot A.; Yang, Yohong; and Posner, Michael I. a) Institute of Neuroinformatics and Lab for Body and Mind, Dalian University of Technology, Dalian 116024, China; b) Department of Psychology, University of Oregon, Eugene, OR 97403; and c) Neuroimaging Research Branch, National Institute on Drug Abuse-Intramural Research Program, Baltimore, MD 21224 (2010). "Short-term meditation induces white matter changes in the anterior cingulate." *PNAS (Proceedings of the National Academy of Sciences of the United States of America)*. Submitted by Posner, Michael I. July 27, 2010. August 16, 2010. pnas.org/content/early/2010/08/10/1011043107.abstract

[12] Jackson, Phil and Delehanty, Hugh (Foreword by Bill Bradley) (2006) Sacred Hoops: Spiritual Lessons of a Hardwood Warrior. Hyperion.

[13] MSNBC: NBCSports: "Kobe to Conan: He had us meditate pre-game." (2009) *NBCSports.com news service*. June 18. 2009.

[14] Medina, Mark. (2010) "Andrew Bynum's meditation proves instrumental in overcoming knee injury." *Los Angeles Times*. Lakers Blog. latimes.com/lakersblog/2010.June 9, 2010.

[15] Lehrer, Jim. (2000). *PBS transcript. Online News Hour*. pbs.org/newshour/bb/sports/jan-june00/jackson_6-16.html. June 16, 2000.

Chapter 14: Reducing the Pain of Disability through Meditation, by Harald Hoermann, M.S.

[1] Antonovsky, Aaron. (1997) *Salutogenese. Zur Entmystifizierung der Gesundheit* (Orig.: (1987) *Unraveling the mystery of health. How people manage stress and stay well*). Tübingen

[2] Steinmann, Ralph Marc. (2008). *Spiritualitaet - Die vierte Dimension der Gesundheit- Eine Einführung aus der Sicht der Gesundheitsfoerderung und Praevention*. Zuerich. (*Spirituality – the Fourth Dimension of Health. An Introduction from a Health Promotion and Preventive Perspective*)

[3] Kabbat-Zinn, Jon. (1991) *Gesund und stressfrei durch Meditation. Das große Buch der Selbstheilung*. Bern (*Healthy and Stress-free with Meditation. The Great Book of Self-healing*)

[4] Singh, Rajinder. (1997) *Empowering Your Soul through Meditation*. Lisle, Illinois: Radiance Publishers.

[5] Singh, Rajinder. (2007) *Inner and Outer Peace through Meditation*. Lisle, Illinois: Radiance Publishers.

[6] Singh, Rajinder. (2011) *Spark of the Divine*. Lisle, Illinois: Radiance Publishers.

[7] Kammerl, Mira. (2010) *Positive Wirkung von Meditation: Eine Studie zu Spiritualitaet, Achtsamkeit, Glueck, Lebenszufriedenheit, Aengstlichkeit, Persoenlichkeit und Meditationstiefe*. Saarbruecken (*Positive Effects of Meditation: A Study of Spirituality, Mindfulness, Happiness, Life Satisfaction, Anxiety, Personality, and Meditation Depth*)

Chapter 15: Meditation and Healing Pain, by James Harris Gruft, M.D., DABPM, FAAPMR

[1] Melzak R., Casey K.L., "Sensory, Motivational and Central Determinants of Pain: A New Conceptual Model." 423-443. Kenshalo D, ed., *The Skin Senses*. Springfield, Illinois: Charles C. Thomas, 1968.

[2] Singh, Rajinder. (1996) *Inner and Outer Peace through Meditation*. Lisle, Illinois: Radiance Publishers, p. 21.

[3] Schachtel, Ernest. (1959) *Metamorphosis*. New York: Basic Books.

[4] Puchalshi et al. (2003) "A Systematic Review of Spiritual and Religious Variables in Palliative Medicine." *American Journal of Hospice and Palliative Care, Hospice Journal, Journal of Palliative Care, and Journal of Pain and Symptom Management.*" Palliative and Supportive Care 2003; 1:7-13.

[5] Gallup G. Jr, Lindsay D. M. (1999) *Surveying the Religious Landscape*. Chicago: University of Chicago Press.

[6] Gallup G. Jr., Castelli J. (1989) *The People's Religion American Faith in the 90s*. New York: McMillan.

[7] Singh Rajinder. (1996) *Inner and Outer Peace through Meditation*. Lisle, Illinois: Radiance Publishers, 30-31.

[8] Campbell J. (1949) *The Hero with a Thousand Faces*. Princeton, New Jersey: Princeton University Press, 385-386.

Radiance Publishers

For information on books by
Radiance Publishers, contact:

Radiance Publishers
1042 Maple Ave.
Lisle, IL 60532

Email: info@radiancepublishers.com